Tradition and the Biological Revolution

The Application of Jewish Law
to the Treatment of the Critically Ill

Tradition and the Biological Revolution

The Application of Jewish Law
to the Treatment of the Critically Ill

DANIEL B. SINCLAIR

EDINBURGH UNIVERSITY PRESS

Edinburgh University Press
22 George Square, Edinburgh

Set in Itek Century Schoolbook
by Carto-Graphics, Edinburgh, and
printed in Great Britain by
Redwood Burn Limited,
Trowbridge, Wilts.

British Library Cataloguing
  in Publication Data
Sinclair, Daniel B.
  Tradition and the biological
    revolution.
1. Jewish law
I. Title
296.1'8
I S B N 0 85224 636 6

CONTENTS

ACKNOWLEDGMENTS

This book originated in a doctoral thesis submitted to the Hebrew University of Jerusalem in 1986. My thanks are due to Prof. S. Shilo who supervised the thesis and read the first draft of the present work. His critical comments were always positive and helpful. I am also in debt to my colleagues at the Institute of Research in Jewish Law at the Hebrew University for helpful comments on many aspects of the topics treated in this book. A debt of gratitude is owed to Prof. M. Elon, Deputy President of the Supreme Court of the State of Israel, who introduced me to the discipline of Jewish law, and to Prof. B. S. Jackson who encouraged me to study it in a wider context. Prof. N. MacCormick provided an opportunity for doing precisely that in the Centre for Criminology and the Social and Philosophical Study of Law at Edinburgh University from 1984-1987. His unfailing enthusiasm for multi-disciplinary studies is warmly acknowledged. My thanks are also extended to Rabbi W. Novick and Mr N. Asher, whose advice and generosity were invaluable in bringing this book to publication. My debt of gratitude to my wife Debbie is enormous. She typed successive drafts of both the thesis and the book, and in the course of doing so, ironed out many a stylistic infelicity. For her constant support for my academic projects, I am deeply grateful. Appendix A originally appeared in Volume 2 of the Jewish Law Association Studies (ed. B.S. Jackson, Atlanta, 1986) and Scholar's Press kindly consented to its publication in this book.

This book is dedicated to Mr and Mrs N. Asher.

Daniel B. Sinclair
Jerusalem, May, 1988

INTRODUCTION

General

This book is concerned with some of the conceptual and moral problems involved in applying Jewish law—*halakhah*[1]—to the treatment of the critically ill in modern medicine. Its starting point is the body of written opinions *(responsa)* composed by modern halakhic authorities on this issue.[2] The analysis of these opinions in Chapter 1 reveals that the authorities are aware of the existence of a conceptual gap between the traditional halakhic category for dealing with the dying and the contemporary problem of terminating the care and treatment of critically ill patients. This analysis is followed by a critical account of the methods by which they seek to bridge this gap and thereby to continue applying the traditional halakhic model to the contemporary situation. Chapter 2 deals with another halakhic category or model which is relevant to a critically ill individual but which has not been applied by halakhists in that context. Chapter 3 is concerned with the ramifications of this category for the issue of sacrificing one life to save another. The final chapter compares these two halakhic categories from both a conceptual and a moral perspective, and a tentative recommendation is made with regard to the choice of category for dealing with the critically ill patient in the context of modern medicine.

The focus of the book is the process by which the traditional categories of Jewish law are applied to radically new situations, hence the title, 'Tradition and the Biological Revolution'. It is hoped that the insights into this process offered in the course of the book will also be useful to students of other traditional legal systems. In this context it is noteworthy that the role of traditionality in understanding modern positivist systems has been emphasised in recent literature.[3] The present study may, therefore, also prove to be of interest to students of jurisprudence in general and not merely to those of overtly traditional systems.

The sub-title indicates that the main issue of this book is the powerful challenge to traditional concepts which has arisen as a result of the revolution in medical science in the last quarter of a century. The main topic dealt with is that of the termination of the life of a critically ill patient when such life is being maintained by sophisticated medical technology. The question of aborting a defective foetus whose condition may now be detected in the early stages of pregnancy is also treated at length. In both cases, recent developments in medical science have fundamentally altered the conceptual and moral framework within which the traditional concepts operate. This area is clearly an extremely fruitful one for study in the context of the process by which *halakhah* adapts to a changing reality.

The first major theoretical issue dealt with in the body of the text is the value of universal moral intuitions in the *halakhah* governing questions of life and death. This issue arises in three contexts. The first is the development of a halakhic policy for dealing with perpetrators of violent crimes who are not subject to the ordinary course of criminal justice. The term 'policy' is apposite in this context since the underlying issue is the effect upon the moral standards of society of leaving such crimes unpunished.[4] A fundamental feature of this policy is the universal moral intuition that any form of bloodshed is a heinous offence for which there must be both a proscription and a penalty within the halakhic framework. The chief architect of this policy is Moses Maimonides, the renowned medieval codifier and philosopher. Maimonides's skilful deployment of traditional sources and moral intuitions is discussed at length in Chapter 2. The ramifications of this policy for the treatment of the critically ill and the weight to be attached to competing moral intuitions arising as a result of the contemporary revolution in the care of the terminal patient constitute the focus of Chapters 3 and 4. A critical study of the Maimonidean model of halakhic policy in this area and its relationship to theories of the juristic development of the *halakhah* is reserved for the last section of the book.

The second context in which the subject of general morality arises is in the criticism of legal doctrine. One instance of such criticism is the discussion of the traditional model for the care of the dying in the first section of Chapter 4. Another instance in the same section is the comparison of halakhic categories relevant to the treatment of the critically ill. Moral intuitions of a universal nature also provide the basis for the critical comparison made at the end of Chapter 3 between the doctrine of necessity as a defence to a murder charge in the common law and the halakhic principle that a non-viable life may be sacrificed for the sake of a viable one. The justification for using general morality as a critical criterion in relation to a halakhic issue is that it is recognised as such by Jewish law in the context of questions of life and death. This claim is made at length in Chapter 2.

The third context in which the issue of universal morality plays a prominent role is in the discussion of the possibility of recognising human suffering as a value in halakhic decisions regarding the critically ill. In this context, the question of whether the *halakhah* in this area grants any authority to conventional moral intuitions is addressed, and a tentative recommendation regarding the weight of suffering as a factor in terminating treatment is made. The bulk of this discussion is to be found in the final section.

The second principal theoretical point explored in this book is the nature of the reasoning employed by halakhic authorities in dealing with radically new objective situations. This issue is the subject of a vast literature in general jurisprudence,[5] and a survey of all the relevant material is clearly beyond the scope of this book. Instead, the focus will be confined to the issue at hand, and in particular, the balance between halakhic policy and halakhic categories in relation to the critically ill. The question of the extent to which halakhic categories are capable of yielding sufficiently developed principles for the resolution of controversial issues in this field is examined at length in both the final chapter and the first appendix. This appendix is devoted to the debate between two outstanding modern halakhic authorities in the field of medical law on the question of aborting a foetus suffering from Tay–Sachs disease. This debate constitutes the major framework for the discussion of legal reasoning in the final chapter.

The book concludes with another appendix of a comparative nature which deals with the current legal position regarding the disconnection of an artificial respirator in the case of a critically ill person.

Preliminary Remarks

The first point which must be made is that in Jewish law a person
does not have the right to dispose of his body purely in accordance
with his wishes:[6] man does not possess absolute title to his life or
his body.[7] As a result of this principle, the issue of the extent to
which the wishes of the patient in question are relevant to the
termination of his treatment does not figure in the body of this text.
There is no right to die in Jewish law, and, hence, devices such as
the 'living will' adopted in various American legislations are
irrelevant to the present study.[8] Suicide is regarded as a crime in
Jewish law.[9] One of the reasons advanced for this is that by taking
his own life, a person denies the divine ownership of his body and
his soul.[10] There are circumstances in which a person is required to
end his life or allow it to be taken, but these are confined to acts of
martyrdom, which are mandatory in cases involving the three
cardinal offences of idolatry, adultery, and murder.[11] Pain and
suffering *per se* would not, therefore, appear to constitute valid
grounds for terminating a person's life, and even according to the
minority view that suicide might be justified in such circumstances,[12]
the critically ill patient with which this book is concerned is
inevitably dependent upon others for all his treatment, including
the termination of such treatment.

This brings us to the second point, namely the nature of the
critical illness mentioned in the subtitle. Since the aim of the book
is to deal with the revolutionary aspects of terminal illness, two
main cases are considered under the rubric of critical illness. The
first is a general condition in which the individual concerned is no
longer capable of independent physical functioning. This state is
typified by the celebrated case of Karen Quinlan, in which the
Supreme Court of New Jersey issued a declaratory judgement to
the effect that hospital staff could disconnect an artificial
respirator from a comatose patient in a persistent vegetative
condition.[13] The second case is that of a specific fatal disease such
as cancer. In both cases, modern medicine has radically altered the
nature of these conditions by its ability to extend minimal
physiological functioning for an indefinite period of time. This
situation provides a unique opportunity for the testing of halakhic
categories and policies in the light of a changing reality. It is,
therefore, not a particular medical condition which is at issue here
but the general problem of the changing face of death and its

evolution from an event to a process.[14] Consequently, the clinical aspects of terminal disease receive only a brief mention in the text, in so far as they are relevant to the discussion of the halakhic models in question. It is not the aim of this work to provide a medical handbook for determining the point at which care and treatment may be terminated according to Jewish law.

A final remark concerns the use of Hebrew terms in the text. The vast majority of these terms refer to works on Jewish law, and their significance in the developmental structure and normative hierarchy of the *halakhah* is indicated in the following section of this Introduction. The sources referred to in the footnotes are of a more specialised nature, but the significance of the literary genre to which they belong is also indicated in the next section. A list of all post-Talmudic sources together with their authors appears at the conclusion of the present work. The few Hebrew terms referring to legal concepts used in this book are the subject of analysis in the body of the text and are fully explained in the contexts in which they occur.

Introductory Remarks on the Structure of Jewish Law[15]

The basic text in any halakhic discussion is the Babylonian *Talmud*. This work, the bulk of which was redacted in the fifth century, constitutes the authoritative compilation of the written and oral traditions of Jewish law. All subsequent legal works are devoted to the explication of the *Talmud*. Commentaries such as that of R. Solomon b. Isaac, commonly known by the acronym Rashi (1040–1105) explain the text of the *Talmud* and make it accessible to the student; Novellae such as those of the *Tosafot* or Glossators (eleventh to thirteenth centuries in France and Germany) are concerned with the development of legal concepts as a result of an integrated view of the whole *Talmud*. Codes such as the *Mishneh Torah* of Moses Maimonides, known as the Rambam (1135–1204) are devoted to the authoritative presentation of Talmudic law in the light of the commentaries and novellae of any particular generation. To these literary genres ought to be added the *responsa*, which are decisions by leading halakhists on difficult or unusual cases. Most of the *responsa* referred to in this book are from the modern period, and hence, contain lengthy and elaborate justifications of the decision given on the issue in question.

The major code of Jewish law is the *Shulhan Arukh,* which was compiled by R. Joseph Karo (1488–1575) and first appeared in Venice in 1564–5. This code became the universally accepted framework for the establishment of the *halakhah,* and its decisions are binding. Many of the issues dealt with in the present study are not, however, included in the *Shulhan Arukh* or its super-commentaries. This is hardly surprising in the light of their contemporary nature. It is to the *Talmud,* therefore, that our attention must be directed in order to resolve the problems arising out of the biological revolution in the modern era. Since the literary medium for dealing with contemporary issues in the Rabbinic world is that of the *responsum,* much of the analysis in the following chapters is devoted to *responsa,* and particularly those of modern authorities. In the absence of a definitive code of Jewish medical law, the *responsa* represent the authoritative halakhic position on such matters.

It is important to note two fundamentally different approaches to the codification of Jewish law. The first, represented by Maimonides, includes the moral and homiletical elements of Judaism in the context of the *halakhah.* The second, typified by R. Joseph Karo, does not. In the final analysis, it was R. Karo's *Shulhan Arukh,* with its faithful adherence to Talmudic form and style, which became the binding compilation of *halakhah.* Maimonides's genius for synthesis notwithstanding, the traditional type of codification prevailed. In the last section of the book, it will be argued that a similar tension exists concerning the issue of the critically ill patient. In Maimonides's *Mishneh Torah,* this issue is treated from a strongly moralistic perspective. This perspective is absent in the *Shulhan Arukh.* Modern authorities take up conflicting positions based upon these two variant approaches to *halakhah.* In this respect, a theory of the structure of *halakhah* is also relevant to its practical application in the context of contemporary halakhic bioethics.

Notes
1. The adjectival form is halakhic. The following general works on the Jewish legal system in the English language may be singled out: Z. Hayyes, *The Student's Guide Through the Talmud,* trans. J. Shachter, (New York, 1960), chs. 1–16; D. Feldman, *Marital Relations, Birth Control and Abortion in Jewish Law* (New York, 1974), ch. 1; *The Principles of Jewish Law,* ed. M. Elon (Jerusalem, 1974).

2. The *responsa* literature is the most dynamic aspect of Jewish law, and is particularly significant in the field of medical matters. On *responsa* in general, see: *Encyclopaedia Judaica* 13, p.83 s.v. *responsa;* S. Freehof, *The Responsa Literature* (Philadephia, 1985), chs. 1–2; Y. Cahana, 'The codified decision and the responsum' (Heb.), Bar-Ilan 1 (1963) 274; B. Lifshitz, 'The legal status of the responsa literature' (Heb.), *Shenaton Hamishpat Haivri* 9–10 (5742–3) 265.

3. See M. Krygier, 'Law as tradition', forthcoming in *Law and Philosophy* 5 (1986); 'Julius Stone: Leeways of choice, legal tradition and the declaratory theory of law', forthcoming in *University of New South Wales Law Journal* and the *Bulletin of the Australian Society for Legal Philosophy.*

4. See R. Dworkin, *Taking Rights Seriously* (London, 1981), pp82ff.

5. The following works on the nature of judicial reasoning are particularly noteworthy: B. Cardozo, *The Nature of the Judicial Process* (New Haven, 1921); J. Stone, *Legal Systems and Lawyers' Reasoning* (London, 1964); E. Levi, *An Introduction to Legal Reasoning* (Chicago, 1949); R. Wasserstrom, *The Judicial Decision* (Stanford, 1961); N. McCormick, *Legal Reasoning and Legal Theory* (Oxford, 1978).

6. See the sources cited in A. Avraham, *Lev Avraham* 2 (Jerusalem, 5738) 133, n.3.

7. J. Bleich, 'The Quinlan case: A Jewish perspective, in *Jewish Bioethics,* ed. F. Rosner, D. Bleich (New York, 1979) p.270.

8. See Appendix B.

9. See Elon (ed.), *Op. cit.,* p.477; F. Rosner, 'Suicide in Jewish law' in *Rosner and Bleich, op. cit.* p.325.

10. Rosner, *op. cit.,* 327.

11. See *Sanh.* 74a; Rosner, *op. cit.*

12. See *Resp, Besamin Rosh* no. 345. Also see I. Rosenbaum, The *Holocaust and Halakhah* (New York, 1976), p.35 for the application of this view during the Holocaust period.

13. *In the Matter of Karen Quinlan* (1976) 70 NJ 355 A 2d 651.

14. P. Aries, *Western Attitudes Towards Death from the Middle Ages to the Present* (Baltimore, 1974), p.88; D. Walton, *On Defining Death* (Montreal, 1979).

15. For a detailed presentation see the sources in n.1. The purpose of these remarks is merely to provide a very brief outline.

1

THE DISTINCTION BETWEEN PRECIPITATING THE DEATH OF A *GOSES* (DYING INDIVIDUAL) AND REMOVING AN IMPEDIMENT

The model for the treatment of the dying in the *Talmud*[1] and the *Shulhan Arukh*[2] is the *goses,* i.e. a person in his death throes. Typical symptoms of this condition, which is known as *gesisah,* are constriction of the chest cavity,[3] accumulation of saliva in the throat,[4] and the emission of a death rattle.[5] According to the *Talmud,* a *goses* is considered a living person in all respects.[6] All legal acts performed by a *goses* are valid, provided that he is lucid and possesses sufficient physical ability to communicate his intentions.[7] No interference with a *goses* is permitted until death is firmly established, and the *Talmud* states that 'one who shuts the eyes of a *goses* is considered as if he had shed his blood'.[8] No preparations for the burial of a *goses* may be undertaken before death lest the knowledge of such activities hastens expiry.[9]

It is presumed that a *goses* will die within a short time of the onset of his condition, and in the *halakhah* this period is fixed at three days.[10] The presumption of death, however, is not an absolute one. Hence, although it is a well-established rule that a person ought to begin mourning rites three days after being informed that a close relative has become a *goses,*[11] the wife of a *goses* is not allowed to remarry merely upon the basis of her husband's condition. For the wife to remarry evidence of the husband's death is always required, since he may belong to the minority of *gosesim* who do, in fact, survive, and the consequences of permitting a woman to remarry when her husband is still alive are extremely grave.[12] In the case of mourning rites, the consequences of applying the presumption of death within three days of the onset of *gesisah* are not unduly serious, hence the application of the presumption in that case.[13]

Most significant is the fact that in Jewish criminal law, the murderer of a *goses* is liable to the death penalty.[14] In this regard, the *goses* is certainly a living person in all respects. The killer of a *terefah* (a person suffering from a fatal disease) is, however, exempt from the death penalty.[15] The fundamental distinction which underlies this difference is that the death of a *terefah* is inevitable, whereas that of a *goses* is not. The murderer of a *terefah* escapes the death penalty since 'his victim is already dead'.[16] In the light of this difference, the *Talmud* distinguishes between two types of *goses*. The first is the *goses* 'at the hands of heaven', i.e. a person reduced to his condition by natural causes. The other is a *goses* 'at the hands of man', i.e. one whose condition was brought about as a result of human action.[17] The question is then raised concerning the penalty for killing a *goses* at the hands of man, and the conclusion is that his killer is not liable to the death penalty.[18] Only the killer of a person suffering from natural death throes is liable to capital punishment. Victims of disease or accident are excluded from the *goses* category as far as capital punishment is concerned.

The major characteristic of the process of *gesisah* which emerges from this survey is its naturalness. The Talmudic *goses* is still capable of instructing those around him and of performing various legal acts. He is not suffering from any manifest fatal disease or wound and may, in fact, survive. The *goses* category clearly reflects the traditional death-bed, with the dying person presiding over a ritual ceremony amidst his assembled relatives and friends.[19] This is the natural context of the laws of the *goses,* and it is against this background that these laws were formulated in the Talmudic and post-Talmudic periods.

An important distinction in relation to the treatment of the *goses* was developed in the Middle Ages. This distinction first appears in the *Sefer Hasidim,* a compendium of teachings of the medieval pietist sect known as the *Hasidei Ashkenaz:*[20]

> Death is not to be delayed, e.g. if there is a woodchopper in the vicinity of the *goses* and the soul is thereby prevented from emerging, the chopper may be removed. Salt is not to be put on the tongue of the *goses* in order to keep him alive.[21] If a *goses* claims that he cannot die unless he is transported to another place, he is not to be removed.[22]

The basic distinction in the above extract is between removing an impediment to death, which is permitted, and precipitating death, which is not. This distinction became the subject of increasingly sophisticated analysis, and was eventually incorporated into the glosses of R. Isserless on the *Shulhan Arukh*.[23] However, it is not only on a normative level that this distinction is a significant one. From the various discussions of this passage in the *Sefer Hasidim* in halakhic literature, it is clear that Jewish communities developed various practices in relation to the treatment of the dying which necessitated distinctions of this type. Noteworthy in this respect are the comments of R. Joshua Boaz, a sixteenth-century Italian scholar who observes that in his youth he had strenuously opposed the widespread custom of removing pillows made of bird feathers from the *goses*. This custom arose from the belief, popular amongst Jews and Christians alike, that these feathers prevented the emergence of the soul.[24] It was, however, sanctioned by R. Boaz's teachers, and his protestations were therefore to no avail.[25] There was, nevertheless, little doubt in R. Boaz's mind that the physical interference involved in removing the pillow from under the head of the *goses* was tantamount to transporting him and, hence, forbidden.[26] He also mentions another prevalent custom of which he disapproved, namely placing the keys of the synagogue under the head of the *goses* in order to precipitate death. Other authorities, however, argued that these practices were indeed sanctioned by the *Sefer Hasidim* as long as they did not involve any rough treatment of the *goses*.[27] Clearly, a certain degree of tension existed between folk practice and the law in this area, and this tension is reflected in the halakhic literature of the period.

R. Moses Isserless incorporated the distinction between removing an impediment and precipitating death into his glosses on the *Shulhan Arukh*[28] in the following terms:

> It is forbidden to hasten death, e.g. if a person is undergoing prolonged death throes and his soul cannot depart, it is prohibited to remove the pillow or cushion from underneath him following the popular belief that the feathers of certain birds contained in the pillow or cushion may prevent the soul from departing. The *goses* may not be moved, nor may the keys of the Synagogue be placed under his head in order to facilitate the departure of his soul. If, however, there is anything which causes a hindrance to the departure of the soul, e.g. the presence near the house of a knocking sound such as the chopping of wood, or if there is salt on the tongue, and

these hinder the soul's departure, then they may be removed, since there is no act involved in this at all, merely the removal of an impediment.[29]

One of the problems arising out of this formulation is the apparently arbitrary distinction between salt on the tongue, which may be removed, and pillows, which may not. One possible explanation is that the salt may be disposed of without any substantial physical contact with the *goses,* which is not the case with regard to the pillow.[30] Another authority maintains that the salt may be taken away since it ought not to have been placed on the tongue of the *goses* in the first place.[31] Yet another explanation of R. Isserless's distinction between salt and pillows is offered by his disciple, R. Mordekhai Jaffe. According to R. Jaffe, pillow removal actively precipitates death in a manner similar to the effect of placing the synagogue keys under the head of the *goses.* In R. Jaffe's view, therefore, physical contact with the *goses* is not forbidden unless the action in question also precipitates his death.[32]

In any case, R. Isserless's prohibition on the removal of pillows was not universally accepted. In the following century, R. Hayyim Benveniste[33] specifically permitted this practice in terms identical to those employed by the critics of R. Boaz's uncompromising stand against it. According to R. Benveniste, any impediment may be removed irrespective of any physical contact with the *goses* which such a removal might involve. The *goses* may not, however, be transported from one place to another, since there is nothing 'outside his body preventing death', i.e. transportation does not constitute the removal of an impediment. In this view, therefore, all external influences prolonging the life of the *goses* are considered impediments and may be removed at the time of the emergence of the soul. It is noteworthy that R. Benveniste also mentions the widespread nature of this practice and its endorsement by previous authorities. Unlike R. Boaz, however, he experiences no difficulty in reconciling these aspects of reality with the relevant legal texts.

With modern developments in this area of medical treatment the line between precipitating death and removing an impediment has become increasingly difficult to draw in practice. The major reason for this difficulty is the changes which have taken place as a result of the biological revolution in the treatment of the dying. Instead of the traditional scene of the dying individual surrounded by his relatives and friends, the modern halakhist must deal with a patient in a hospital room, whose death must be impeded, in theory at any rate, by all those treating him. The fundamental question, therefore, is the point at which medical treatment may in fact be terminated. Now, this treatment includes basic physiological activities such as respiration and nutrition. Under which circumstances, if any, may such treatment be classified as an impediment and, hence, terminated? Clearly, there exists a wide conceptual gap between the removal of a woodchopper and, for example, the disconnection of an artificial respirator. As a result of this gap, very few modern Rabbinical authorities have been prepared to make a simple analogy between the two and issue an outright permission to disconnect the respirator whenever *gesisah* is established.[34] Instead, two different approaches to the problem of this conceptual gap may be detected in modern halakhic literature on the issue of the treatment of the dying.

One method of dealing with this gap is to shift the emphasis to the condition of the dying person rather than the nature of the act. Once a certain stage in the process of *gesisah* is reached, all treatment is considered as an impediment to death and must be terminated. The chief exponent of this view is R. Eliezer Waldenburg, a contemporary authority on medical matters in Jewish law. According to R. Waldenburg, there are two phases in the process of *gesisah*.[35] The first phase is the one referred to in the *halakhah,* and in relation to which the classical distinction between different types of acts is made. This is also the phase in which recovery is a faint possibility. The second and final phase, however, is a result of modern technology: it is the twilight zone between life and death, charac- terised by the irreversible cessation of all capacity for independent life. At this stage, all forms of treatment are to be discontinued. R. Waldenburg attempts to find support for his position in earlier authorities,[36] but this support is hardly unqualified. Indeed, it is difficult to avoid the conclusion that R. Waldenburg's main concern is to focus halakhic attention upon the question of defining death for the purposes of terminating all life-supporting treatment rather than upon the distinction between removing an impediment and precipitating death. The extent to which R. Waldenburg succeeded in this endeavour may be gauged from the fact that the physician whose question prompted R. Waldenburg's *responsum* observed that, in the final analysis, all he had done was to rule that there is no obligation to continue treating a patient who was clinically dead, since final phase *gesisah* consists of the loss of all independent capacity in both heart and brain.[37] R. Waldenburg's reply to this objection was to admit that this was indeed the case, and that the main point of his *responsum* was to preclude the argument that a patient bereft of detectable independent life ought to be treated on the grounds that he might still possess some undetected independent capacity.[38] It is therefore evident that R. Waldenburg's attempt to overcome the conceptual constraints of the *goses* category by distinguishing between two phases of *gesisah* is both a departure from previous doctrine and of questionable practical value.

Other modern authorities deal with this conceptual problem by removing the maintenance of all basic physiological functions such as nutrition and respiration from the category of impediments to death. This view is often accompanied by the observation that the definition of *gesisah* is not necessarily applicable to a terminally ill patient who may, with constant medical attention, be able to live for an indeterminate period of time.[39] According to this view, the sole significance of the permission to remove an impediment for modern medicine is that a critically ill patient need not receive aggressive life-prolonging treatment. Both artificial respiration and intravenous feeding must be maintained until the establishment of death. This approach empties the notion of impediment removal of almost all its content and seems to reflect a purely moral position regarding the treatment of the dying.[40] In this respect, the conceptual gap has indeed been bridged, but in an untraditional fashion, i.e. a general theory of the sanctity of life has replaced the legal doctrine of the *goses*.[41]

The development of such a general theory is indeed the aim of the modern discipline of bioethics. A leading bioethicist, however, has observed that the chances of propounding such a theory and of arriving at practical solutions are very slim in the pluralistic societies of contemporary times. In his view, traditional systems such as Jewish law are far more capable of providing such solutions since they possess both the intellectual apparatus and the necessary social uniformity for their provision.[42] In the light of the above observations, however, it would seem that Jewish law is in no better shape than general bioethics, since it, too, is ultimately dependent upon a general philosophy of the treatment of the dying rather than upon any particular legal doctrine. This trend is particularly evident in the view which maintains that the critically ill patient of modern medicine is not to be classified as a *goses* for the purpose of applying the distinction between removing an impediment and precipitating death. A contemporary Jewish bioethic would seem to be as elusive as a general one, and even on a purely legal level there is disagreement amongst contemporary authorities regarding the removal of an artificial respirator and the cessation of intravenous feeding. Moreover, such an approach, if it were institutionalised, would constitute a radical break with traditional Judaism, which regards the law as the sole authority for dealing with the problems of life.[43]

In fact, there is another category within Jewish legal doctrine which may be more effective in tackling the problems raised by prolonging the lives of the critically ill. This is the category of *terefah*, and it is to this category that the following chapters are devoted. In addition to an outline of the *terefah* in Jewish law, particular attention will be paid to the significance of this category for determining the criminal nature of terminating the life of a critically ill patient, and the question of sacrificing one life for the sake of saving another.

Notes

1. *Sem.* ch.1; *Shab.* 151b.
2. *Shulhan Arukh, Yoreh Deah* 339.
3. R. Moses Isserless, *Shulhan Arukh, Even Haezer* 121:7.
4. *Tosafot Yom Tov, Arak.* 1:3.
5. Maimonides, *Commentary to the Mishnah, Arak.* 1:3; *Tiferet Yisrael, Arak.* 1-3; *Arukh Hashalem s.v. gasas,* no.2. According to a modern physician, the traditional criteria of *gesisah* correspond to the destruction of the gag reflex in the dying process: see A. Dagi, 'The paradox of euthanasia', *Judaism* 23 (1975), 164.
6. *Sem.* 1:1. For a general survey of the legal status of the *goses* in the Talmud, see *Encyclopaedia Talmudit* 5, p.393.
7. See *Gitt.* 70b; *Tur, Even Haezer* 121; *Bah, Even Haezer* 121; *Bet Yosef, Even Haezer* 121; *Shulhan Arukh, Even Haezer* 121:7; *Kidd.* 78b.
8. *Sem.* 1:2-7; *Shab.* 151b.
9. Nahmanides, *Torat Haadam, Inyan Hapetirah, s.v. klalo shel davar;* Rema, *Shulhan Arukh, Yoreh Deah* 339.
10. *Gitt.* 28a; *Perishah, Tur, Yoreh Deah* 339:5 and see n. 11 below.
11. Rosh, *M. Kat.* 3:97; Moredekhai, *M. Kat.* 864; *Tur, Yoreh Deah* 339; *Shulhan Arukh, Yoreh Deah* 339:2.
12. *Tosafot, Yeb.* 120b, *s.v. lemimra; Tosafot, Yeb.* 36b, *s.v. ha; Tosafot, Bekh.* 20b, *s.v. helev;* Rosh, *Bekh.* 3:2; *Pithei Teshuva, Even Haezer* 17:131 and *Yoreh Deah* 339:3; *Resp, Noda Beyehuda* 1, no. 59, cf. *Beth Shmuel, Even Haezer* 17:94.

13. Some authorities maintain that since the presumption of death is not strong enough to permit a woman to remarry, mourning rites ought not to be initiated on its basis: see *Pithei Teshuva, Yoreh Deah* 339:3. However, this is not the accepted view.

14. *Sanh.* 78a; Maimonides, *Hil. Rozeah* 2:7.

15. *Sanh.* 78a; Maimonides, *Hil. Rozeah* 2:8. For the definition and legal status of the *terefah,* see below, ch. 2, p.20.

16. *Yad Remah, Sanh.* 78a; *Minhat Hinukh* no. 34; H. Cohn, 'On the dichotomy of divinity and humanity in Jewish law' in *Euthanasia,* ed. A. Carmi (Berlin, 1984), p.55 and below, ch. 3, p.21.

17. *Sanh.* 78a.

18. Maimonides, *Hil. Rozeah* 2:7, see Cohn, *op. cit.* 56.

19. P. Aries, *Western Attitudes towards Death from the Middle Ages to the Present* (Baltimore, 1974), p.88. Clearly, this description applies to the East in the same way as it does the West.

20. See J. Dan, *Torat Hasod Shel Hasidei Ashkenaz* (Jerusalem, 5726); G. Scholem, *Major Trends in Jewish Mysticism* (New York, 1940), pp.80ff.; I. Baer, 'The religious social tendency of *Sefer Hasidim'* (Heb.), *Zion* 3 (5698); H. Soloveitchik, 'Three themes in *Sefer Hasidim', Association for Jewish Studies Review* 1 (1976), 311. It would appear that this movement had an ambivalent attitude towards the Christian pietist movements of the time, both reacting against them and being influenced by them.

21. See J. Trachtenberg, *Jewish Magic and Superstition* (New York, 1939), p.160. Salt, in particular, was believed to possess magical qualities and could repel demons and evil spirits.

22. *Sefer Hasidim,* ed. R. Margaliot (Jerusalem 5717) no. 723. There are two editions of the *Sefer Hasidim,* one printed in Bologna (1583) and the other found in manuscript in Parma and published in Berlin (1891–4) and Frankfurt (1924). This particular section is identical in all editions, and the present reference is therefore to the standard one. Tradition ascribes the authorship of the whole *Sefer Hasidim* to R. Judah the Hasid (d. 1217), the great teacher of the *Hasidei Ashkenaz.* According to various scholars, however, R. Eliezer of Worms, R. Judah's most prominent disciple, was the author of some passages in *Sefer Hasidim,* and was probably its editor. On the subject of the authorship of *Sefer Hasidim,* see the works cited in n.3 above, and J. Wistenetzki and J. Friemann (eds), *Sefer Hasidim* (Frankfurt, 1924). It is noteworthy that from the fifteenth century onwards, the *Sefer Hasidim* was also used by writers of *halakhah* as an authoritative source on the Jewish way of life.

23. *Yoreh Deah* 339:1.

24. According to Trachtenberg, op. cit., p.160, the removal of such pillows was an anti-demonic practice prevalent in the Middle Ages. Trachtenberg's assertion that such superstitions were common to Christians and Jews in this period is borne out by the existence of a Christian work devoted entirely to the evils of the practice of removing pillows made of the feathers of certain birds from beneath the heads of the dying. In his *De Pulvineri Morientibus Non Subtrahendo* (Jena, 1678), Caspar Questelius fulminates against this 'particularly detestable' practice which 'although frequently practised is quite obnoxious and inexcusable' (Preface). From Questelius's work, it would appear that the practice was an ancient one, and even

as late as the seventeenth century, it was still necessary to rebut it in the following terms:

> Even though such a custom had existed for a thousand years, whose origin, however, having been gradually introduced, is uncertain, nonetheless, if we have grasped its inherent wickedness, even now it is still a convenient time to correct it, and there is a necessity to do so. (1:7)

Clearly, practices of this nature relating to the treatment of the dying were widespread amongst Jewish and Christian societies, and it is particularly noteworthy that the custom of removing pillows, which is the subject of a debate amongst Jewish scholars in the fifteenth to seventeenth centuries, also figures in the above-mentioned Christian dissertation as a matter of conflict between religious tradition and general practice.

25. *Shiltei Hagiborim, M. Kat.* ch.3 (16b, sec. 4).
26. Cf. *Derishah, Tur, Yoreh Deah* 339. According to this authority, R. Boaz would permit the removal of a pillow if it were done gently, since the act of removal *per se* does not precipitate death.
27. See n.26 above.
28. One of R. Moses Isserless's main objects in these glosses was the incorporation of Ashkenazic traditions into the primarily Shephardic *Shulhan Arukh*. It is therefore to be expected that a distinction originating from the *Hasidei Ashkenaz* would be incorporated into the *Shulhan Arukh* by R. Isserless: see M. Elon, *Hamishpat Haivri* (Jerusalem, 5733) 1126.
29. *Shulhan Arukh, Yoreh Deah* 339:1.
30. *Siftei Kohen, Yoreh Deah* 339:7.
31. *Beth Lehem Yehuda, Yoreh Deah* 339:1. Nevertheless, care must be taken in order to ensure that the *goses* is not jolted in the course of the removal. In this respect, there is little difference between this explanation and the previous one, cf. *Resp. Ziz Eliezer* 13 no. 89 and 14 no. 80.
32. *Levush Mordekhai, Yoreh Deah* 339:1.
33. *Sheirei Knesset Hagedolah, Tur, Yoreh Deah, Hil. Bikkur Holim* 339:4.
34. See R. Hayyim Halevi, 'Disconnecting a terminal patient from an artificial respirator' (Heb.) *Tehumin* 2 (5741) 304; R. Barukh Rabinowitz, 'A symposium on the determination of death and organ transplantation' (Heb.), *Sefer Assia*, ed. A. Steinberg (Jerusalem, 5739) 197.
35. *Resp. Ziz Eliezer* 13 no. 89, and 14 nos 80, 81. See also *Resp. Lev Aryeh* 2 no. 36.
36. R. Waldenburg derives the notion of irreversible loss of capacity for independent physical functioning from the somewhat obscure term 'not because of his body' used by R. Jehiel Epstein *(Arukh Hashulhan, Yoreh Deah* 339:4) in defining an impediment to death. The division between the stages of *gesisah* is traced to R. Joseph Nathanson *(Divrei Saul, Yoreh Deah, Hilkhot Avelut* 194). In neither case is there particularly convincing evidence of support for R. Waldenburg's analysis.
37. *Resp. Ziz Eliezer* 14 nos 80, 81.
38. In elaborating this issue, R. Waldenburg cites *Resp. Hatam Sofer, Yoreh Deah* no. 338 in which the principle that Jewish law does not recognise any definition of death other than those recognised by the

halakhah is presented in most unequivocal terms by R. Moses Sofer
in the eighteenth century. The *responsum* was written in reply to
suggested legislation that burial may be delayed until death could be
established by means such as changes in the colour and composition
of the corpse. R. Sofer also states in no uncertain terms that Jewish
law does not recognise the possibility that someone may be buried
alive as a grounds for delaying interment beyond the time stipulated
by the *halakhah*. In this area, statistical regularity is the crucial
factor: see also Resp. Hayyim Sha'al 2 no. 25; *Resp. Maharaz Hayyes*
no. 52. On this basis. R. Waldenburg argues, it is forbidden to
maintain artificial respiration on the grounds that the patient may
yet possess some undetected source of independent life.

39. *Resp. Nezer Matai* no. 30; *Resp. Beth Avi* 2 no. 153; *Resp. Iggrot
     Moshe, Hoshen Mishpat* 2 no. 73; R. Moses Wolner, 'The physician's
     rights and jurisdiction' (Heb.), Hatorah Vehamedinah 7–8 (5716–7)
     353; R. Immanuel Jakobowitz, 'Concerning the possibility of permitting
     the precipitation of the death of a fatally-ill patient in severe pain'
     (Heb.), *Hapardes* 31 (5717) 18; R. Nissan Telushkin, 'The authority of
     man over his own life in the light of the *halakhah*' (Heb.), *Or
     Hamizrah* 8 (5721) 24; R. Simha Kook, 'Killing a suffering individual'
     (Heb.), *Torah Shebal Peh* 18 (5736) 87; R. David Bleich, 'Ethico-
     halakhic considerations in the practice of medicine', *Dine Israel* 7
     (1976); 'The Quinlan case: A Jewish perspective', in Jewish Bioethics,
     ed. F. Rosner, D. Bleich, (New York, 1979), p.266; A. Steinberg,
     'Mercy-killing in the light of the halakhah' (Heb.), *Sefer Assia,* ed.
     A. Steinberg (Jerusalem, 5743) 451, cf. *Resp. Lev Aryeh* 2 no. 36;
     Halevi, *op. cit.;* Rabinowitz, *op. cit.*

40. This contention is supported by the high level of homiletical material
     in the *responsa,* and many of the articles, cited in n. 39 above.

41. See especially *Resp. Nezer Matai* no. 30; Wolner, *op. cit.;* Bleich, *op.
     cit.;* and see the remarks of R. Hayyim Zimmerman, 'Life as a relative
     concept in *halakhah'*, *Intercom* 11 (1970), 3.

42. D. Callahan, 'Bioethics as a discipline', in *Biomedical Ethics and the
     Law,* ed. J. Humber, R. Almedar (New York, 1977), p.10. The features
     which Callahan highlights in this respect are an exhaustive body of
     well-established and highly refined primary and secondary principles,
     and a long history of sophisticated casuistic reasoning.

43. See A. Lichtenstein, 'Does Jewish tradition recognize an ethic
     independent of *halakhah?',* in *Contemporary Jewish Ethics,* ed. M.
     Kellner (New York, 1978), p.102. One of the claims advanced by
     Lichtenstein is that general moral principles in Judaism are derived
     from the 'penumbra of commandments'. He also observes that
     'relation to a fundamental law, which posits frontiers and points a
     direction, is obviously essential' (p.117). There is a striking similarity
     between this argument and the one advanced by N. MacCormick in
     relation to the development of legal principles from clusters of
     existing legal rules: see his *Legal Reasoning and Legal Theory*
     (Oxford, 1978), ch.7.

2

HUMAN *TARFUT* (FATAL CONDITION) AND THE EXEMPTION OF THE KILLER OF A *TEREFAH* (SUFFERER OF A FATAL DISEASE) FROM CAPITAL PUNISHMENT

The Terefah Category

Although the category upon which most attention has been focused in the context of the biological revolution in the field of the treatment of the dying is that of the *goses,* there is another Talmudic category which is relevant to this topic, known as the *terefah.* In the course of the following chapters, it will be argued that this is the category which contains the solutions for some of the most pressing issues in contemporary medical law, namely, the correct approach to the criminal nature of terminating the life of a critically ill patient, and the principles underlying the allocation of scarce medical resources. In arguing that the best approach to current bioethical issues is the development of an existing category within the legal tradition of Judaism rather than a general philosophy of life and death drawn from either received or conventional morality, a statement is also being made in favour of a particular theory of juristic development. This is the theory that such development takes place within traditional categories rather than general philosophies, and that the categories in question possess the capacity for such development. It is to this theory that much of the final chapter of the book is devoted.

The term *terefah* is a familiar one in the context of Jewish dietary laws where it refers to an animal suffering from a fatal organic defect, e.g. a pierced windpipe or gullet.[1] Such an animal may not be eaten, even if it is slaughtered in the prescribed manner. The defects constituting animal *tarfut* (fatal condition) are specified in the *Talmud* and Codes, and scientific evidence as to whether or not they are actually fatal is completely irrelevant.[2] It is presumed that a *terefah* animal will die within twelve months; hence, a doubtful case may be consumed if it survives for a longer period.[3] Survival of an established *terefah* for more than a year is ascribed to supernatural forces.[4]

In the human context, however, the meaning of the term *terefah* is much less precise. The classical definition is provided by Maimonides in relation to the exemption of the killer of a *terefah* person from capital punishment on the grounds that the victim is 'already dead'.[5] Maimonides's definition runs as follows: 'it is known for certain that he had a fatal organic disease and physicians say that his disease is incurable by human agency, and that he would have died of it even if he had not been killed in another way.[6] Thus, in direct contrast to an animal *terefah,* the human *terefah* is defined on the basis of medical evidence.[7] The primacy of such evidence in the establishment of human *tarfut* (the condition of being a *terefah)* was reiterated in a definitive fashion by R. Moses Feinstein in a recent *responsum* on various bioethical dilemmas.[8]

It is also noteworthy that according to R. Hayyim Grodzinski, the *terefah* category applies to an internal disease, and not necessarily to an injury sustained as a result of an external blow. According to R. Grodzinski, a person suffering from an internal disease from which, according to his doctors, there is no chance of recovery is classified as a *terefah.*[9] R. Grodzinski maintains that the feature of externality is characteristic of animal rather than human *terefot,* since the former are all visible to the eye of the person inspecting the animal after slaughter. On this basis, therefore, any person suffering from a fatal internal disease may be classified as a *terefah,*[10] and his killer will be exempt from the death penalty provided that there is sufficient medical evidence of the fatal nature of his victim's condition. Since the position regarding the killing of a *terefah* in Jewish law will be dealt with at length in Chapter 3, it is unnecessary to take this issue any further at this point.

The other aspect of the definition of animal *terefot* already mentioned, i.e. the presumption of death within twelve months, is also modified in the context of human beings. According to the *halakhah,* the deserted wife of an established *terefah* may be permitted to remarry since the death of a *terefah* is inevitable and evidence of *tarfut* is, therefore, tantamount to evidence of death.[11] According to the majority of authorities, twelve months must elapse before such permission may be granted, analogous with the presumption regarding animal *terefot*.[12] *Tosafot,* however, maintain that a fundamental physiological difference exists between animals and human beings, with the result that the latter may very well be capable of surviving for a longer period.[13] This does not mean, however, that a *terefah* is capable of living for an indeterminate period of time. *Tosafot* merely observe that the fixed time limit is not applicable in the human context in the same way that it is applied to animal *tarfut*. At the same time, the view of *Tosafot* indicates that the twelve month time limit is not as conclusive in relation to human beings as it is in the context of the dietary laws. On this basis, it is arguable that the application of the category of *terefah* to the critically ill of modern medicine ought not to depend strictly upon the twelve month limit. The main factor in any such categorisation ought to be the inevitability of death as a result of fatal illness, with the element of time constituting an important, but not paramount, element in the determination of that inevitability. The twelve month time limit is not absolute in relation to human beings.[14]

The fundamental concept in the definition of human *tarfut* is, therefore, the inevitability of death. This is also the major distinguishing factor between the categories of *goses* and *terefah*. As such, in describing the legal status of the *terefah,* the expression *gavra katila* (dead man) is often used. This is the rationale underlying the rule that the killer of a *terefah* is legally exempt from capital punishment, since he killed someone who was, in effect, already dead.[15] In contrast to the *goses,* whose status as a living being is generally beyond any doubt, the *terefah* is regarded as a 'dead man' in various branches of the *halakhah*. According to some authorities, a *terefah* son renders his widowed mother liable to a levirate marriage.[16] It has also been suggested that the biblical prohibition on marrying the sister of a living wife does not apply if the latter is a *terefah*.[17] Although these views have not gained general acceptance,[18] the fundamental assumption involved in them, i.e. the non-personhood of the *terefah,* is clearly a well-established principle in Jewish law.

There are, however, at least two cases in which it would appear that the status of the *terefah* as 'dead man' is, in fact, an operative one. The first is that of the exemption of the killer of a *terefah* from capital punishment. Here, the underlying rationale is that the victim would have died in any case, and there is no capital punishment for killing a dead man.[19] The second is the permission given to a woman to remarry on the strength of evidence as to her husband's *tarfut* in a case where he has disappeared. Evidence of *gesisah,* however, would not be sufficient for this purpose.[20] Thus, in both cases, the legal status of the *terefah* clearly reflects the conceptual essence of the human *terefah* as a non-person. It is significant that the *halakhah* does not relate to the *goses* as a non-person in either of these cases. Moreover, a person who murders a *goses* is liable to capital punishment, and evidence of *gesisah* is insufficient to permit remarriage.

The outstanding feature of the category of human *tarfut* for the current debate concerning the treatment of the critically ill is the exemption of the killer of a *terefah* from the death penalty.[21] This feature focuses attention upon the fact that a fatal disease does detract from the legal status of a person, and also introduces a measure of flexibility into the issue of terminating such a life. This is in direct contrast to the category of *goses,* which is based on the premise that a *goses* is like a living person in all respects.[22] Indeed, almost all the laws of the *goses* confirm his living status and, as already observed, can only be appreciated against the background of the domestic death-bed.[23] The *terefah* category adopts a different perspective, (the effects of the critical illness upon a person's legal status) and as such, it is much closer to the current debate on the termination of the life of a critically ill patient.

The Exemption of the Killer of a Terefah from Capital Punishment, and the Invocation of Divine Sanctions

According to the *Talmud,* it is universally accepted that the killer of a *terefah* is not liable to the death penalty for his act.[24] Maimonides formulates the relevant *halakhah* as follows:

> If one kills another who suffers from a fatal organic disease, he is exempt from human law even though the victim ate and drank and walked out on the streets. But every human being is presumed to be healthy, and his murderer must be put to death unless it is known for certain that he had a fatal organic disease.[25]

The reason for the exemption is that capital punishment is not administered if, as in this case, the victim would have died of his disease in any case.[26] Since at the time of his murder a *terefah* is as good as dead,[27] his killer is not subject to the regular sanctions of the criminal law. It must be emphasised that this exemption from legal sanction applies only to the murderer of a *terefah* whose non-viability is an established fact. All other murderers are liable to the death penalty, even if the victim was in his death throes.[28] Exemption of the killer in the case of a *terefah* is, therefore, a result of the principle in Jewish criminal law under which there is no death penalty for the murder of a person whose life would in any case be terminated by a fatal organic disease.

The use of the phrase 'exempt from human law' in Maimonides's formulation of the legal exemption of the killer of a *terefah* from human jurisdiction, however, indicates that he is still subject to divine retribution. The point that exemption from human jurisdiction does not entail exemption from divine punishment is made quite explicitly by Maimonides in relation to indirect homicide and suicide:

> If . . . one hires an assassin to kill another, or sends his slave to kill him,[29] or ties another up and leaves him in front of a lion or another animal and the animal kills him,[30] and similarly if one commits suicide,[31] the rules in each of these cases is that he is a shedder of blood, has committed the crime of murder and is liable to death at the hands of Heaven, but there is no capital punishment.
>
> How do we know that this is the rule? Because Scripture says, 'Whoever sheds man's blood, by man shall his blood be shed' *(Gen.* 9:6) referring to one who commits the murder himself and not through an agent; 'And surely your blood of your lives will I require' *(Gen.* 9:5) referring to suicide; 'At the hand of every beast will I require it' *(Gen.* 9:5) referring to one who places another before a wild animal for it to devour; 'And at the hand of man even at the hand of every man's brother, will I require the life of man' *(Gen.* 9:5) referring to one who hires others to kill someone.[32] In these last three cases, the verb 'require' is used expressly to show that their judgment is reserved for Heaven.[33]

Although there is no capital punishment in these cases, Maimonides provides that the individuals concerned are criminals and are liable to death at the hands of Heaven. Support for this ruling is derived from the exegesis of the biblical passage containing the covenant between God and Noah after the Deluge.

This exegesis[34] provides the basis for the offence of bloodshed in
the pre-Sinaitic system of norms referred to in the Rabbinic
tradition as the Noahide laws.[35]

Now, although the scope of the offence of bloodshed in the
Noahide code is much wider than that of the crime of murder in the
halakhah and does indeed extend to indirect homicide and
suicide,[36] Noahide law on this issue would not seem to be
applicable to Israelites after the giving of the Torah.[37] The
relevance of this exegesis as a justification for a ruling in a halakhic
code is therefore highly questionable. Moreover, even if a link were
to be established between the Noahide offence of bloodshed and
the cases of indirect homicide and suicide in the context of Jewish
law, the discrepancy between the death penalty prescribed for
these actions under Noahide law[38] and the mere invocation of
divine retribution in Maimonides's ruling would still need to be
explained. Maimonides's attempt to justify his ruling in terms of
the biblical exegesis cited above is, therefore, in need of further
explanation.

In order to understand the full significance of Maimonides's
reference to the Noahide offence of bloodshed in the above
citation, it would be useful to begin with an analysis of a passage in
the *Mekhilta Derabbi Yishmael*[39] dealing with the punishment for
killing a heathen in Jewish law. On the basis of scriptural
interpretation, the *Mekhilta* concludes that an Israelite who kills a
heathen is exempt from the death penalty. Scripture specifies that
capital punishment is to be imposed only upon someone who
murders his 'neighbour',[40] and a heathen is not included in that
category. The following objection to this conclusion is then
raised:

> Issi b. Akabyah says: Before the giving of the Torah, we had
> been warned against shedding blood. After the giving of the
> Torah, whereby laws were made stricter, shall they be
> considered lighter? In truth, the Sages said: He is free from
> judgment by the human court, but his judgment is left to
> Heaven.[41]

Issi b. Akabyah begins his critique by observing that before the
giving of the Torah, there was no distinction between Israelites and
heathens with respect to the offence of bloodshed. Any person
found guilty of the crime of homicide was liable to the death
penalty, irrespective of his creed. The point is then made that the

purpose of the Torah was to raise the moral standards of the
Israelites above those required by the Noahide code, i.e. 'laws were
made stricter'. The assumption that the Noahide code constitutes
the moral foundation of the *halakhah* is implicit in the Talmudic
principle that 'there is nothing permitted to an Israelite yet
prohibited to a Noahide'.[42] Indeed, according to R. Nissim
Gerondi, Jewish criminal law does not even come into force unless
the relevant provisions of the Noahide code are fully operative in
the society of the time.[43] The basis for R. Issi b. Akabyah's
objection to the *Mekhilta's* ruling regarding the murder of a
heathen is now clear. If the *halakhah* cannot fall below the standard
set by Noahide law, how can an Israelite who commits murder be
treated more leniently than a Noahide who commits the same
offence?

In their reply to this objection, the Sages clearly imply that they
accept the characterisation of the Noahide offence of bloodshed as
a universal moral standard below which the *halakhah* cannot fall.
According to the Sages, the sole difference between Noahide law
and *halakhah* in this respect is the nature of the penalty for the
offence. Whereas the sanction for bloodshed in Noahide law is
capital punishment, in the *halakhah,* the killer of a non-Jew is
subject to divine jurisdiction. Clearly, the act in question is
recognised as a form of homicide by the *halakhah,* and divine
retribution is invoked with regard to the killing of a heathen as it is
in other cases in which religious and moral norms lack positive legal
sanctions.[44] The reply of the Sages to R. Issi b. Akabyah thus
accepts his premise concerning the relationship between Jewish
and Noahide law, and is indeed incorporated by Maimonides into
his *Mishneh Torah* as follows: ' . . . the heathen with whom we are
not at war . . . it is forbidden to cause[45] their death'.[46] The sanction
of divine retribution would also appear to be the authoritative
halakhic response in a case of this nature.[47]

The reason for the difference in penalties between the two
systems is a matter of speculation, and one of the more interesting
suggestions is that the Sinaitic covenant between God and the
Israelites entailed the rejection of the generally cruel and barbaric
modes of punishment practised in the ancient world.[48] Be that as it
may, the short point is that the invocation of divine punishment for
the killing of a heathen indicates that the Noahide offence of
bloodshed constitutes an integral part of Jewish criminal juris-

prudence and, in substance at least, was not abrogated by the giving of the Torah.

The conceptual basis for Maimonides's ruling in the cases of indirect homicide and suicide is now clear. As already observed, both categories are included in the offence of bloodshed in the Noahide code.[49] The *halakhah,* however, exempts the offenders from the death penalty for the reasons outlined above. Maimonides follows the line of reasoning adopted by the Sages in the *Mekhilta.* First, he cites the scriptural source on the basis of which these acts are proscribed under the Noahide code. This, in turn, provides a basis for the invocation of divine punishment in relation to Israelites guilty of these offences.[50] The invocation of Divine punishment is therefore the result of a general theory regarding the links between the Noahide offence of bloodshed and the jurisprudence of Jewish criminal law.

In his classical commentary on the *Mishneh Torah,*[51] R. Joseph Karo explains that the source for Maimonides's ruling is the Talmudic view that killing by proxy is subject to death at the hands of Heaven.[52] In relation to indirect homicide and suicide, however, he falls back on the Noahide prohibition on bloodshed as the source for Maimonides's position. In this respect, the general theory outlined above is more satisfactory, since it provides a unified explanation for the invocation of divine punishment in all three cases. According to this approach, Maimonides's ruling is based upon an underlying theory regarding the relationship between the Noahide offence and the criminal jurisprudence of Jewish law. Moreover, as will be observed, this link is not confined to those cases in which there is a direct source in Talmudic literature.

Maimonides's implication that the killer of a *terefah* is liable to divine retribution, notwithstanding the fact that he is exempt from human law, may be explained in a similar fashion. In his definition of the offence of bloodshed under Noahide law, Maimonides includes the killing of a *terefah.*[53] According to the *halakhah,* however, the fatal nature of his victim's condition precludes the application of the death penalty to the perpetrator of such an act. Following the above theory, therefore, Maimonides rules that the killer is, in fact, subject to divine jurisdiction.

However, there is an obvious difference between the cases of indirect homicide and suicide on the one hand, and the killing of a *terefah* on the other. Whereas the former are specifically mentioned in the *Midrash* as offences constituting the Noahide prohibition on bloodshed, the latter is not.[54] Indeed, various commentators on the *Mishneh Torah* have been perplexed by the apparent lack of any source for Maimonides's inclusion of the killing of a *terefah* in the list of offences constituting bloodshed in the Noahide code.[55] The question that now arises, therefore, is that of the basis for Maimonides's treatment of the killing of a *terefah* as an act proscribed under Noahide law.

The answer to this question is undoubtedly to be found in the rational character of the Noahide laws in general,[56] and the offence of bloodshed in particular. If it can be demonstrated that the Noahide prohibition on bloodshed extends to any act which reasonably can be identified as the shedding of blood, even if there is no formal source for such an identification, then Maimonides's inclusion of the killing of a *terefah* in the Noahide laws will be vindicated, as will his invocation of divine punishment upon the killer in the context of Jewish criminal law. It is to the examination of this possibility that the following paragraphs are devoted.

The rational nature of the Noahide code as a whole is indicated by Maimonides in his statement that although these laws were commanded by God, reason nevertheless 'inclines to them'.[57] Although Maimonides also writes that a gentile who observes the Noahide laws 'because of the determination of reason is not of the pious of the nations nor of their wise men',[58] it is widely accepted that the printed version of the last phrase is incorrect and should in fact read, 'but of their wise men', in accordance with the version in the Bodleian manuscript of the *Mishneh Torah*.[59] It is also noteworthy that Maimonides makes the point that the purpose of the Noahide laws is a rational one, i.e. 'to prevent the world becoming corrupt'.[60]

For the purposes of the present argument, however, it is sufficient to show that the offence of bloodshed alone constitutes a rational law which must be part of any legal system, including Jewish law, if civilised society is to survive.[61] Support for this contention may, in fact, be derived from the *Talmud* itself, which provides that murder may not be committed even at the cost of a person's own life on the basis of the argument. 'How do you know that your blood is redder? Perhaps the blood of the other person is redder!'[62] This argument, clearly is based on reason alone.[63] It is noteworthy that this rational principle is then used in order to provide the basis for elucidating the same rule with respect to forbidden sexual relations.[64]

The rational element in the crime of homicide in Maimonidean jurisprudence is particularly evident in the following passage from the *Mishneh Torah* in which Maimonides refers to the Talmudic requirement that murderers who escape capital punishment by virtue of a technical defect in the testimony against them are nevertheless severely punished for their deeds:[65]

> For although there are worse [i.e. in the theological sense] crimes than bloodshed, none causes such destruction to civilized society[66] as bloodshed. Not even idolatry, nor immorality, nor the desecration of the Sabbath is the equal of bloodshed.[67]

Maimonides justifies the harsh measures taken against murderers who escape the death penalty on the basis of the rational principle of the preservation of civilised society. It is also noteworthy that Maimonides justifies the whole Noahide code in terms of preventing the world becoming corrupt, and undoubtedly, the offence of bloodshed plays a fundamental role in this justification.[68]

The basis for Maimonides's inclusion of the killing of a *terefah* in the Noahide offence of bloodshed is now evident. It is derived from both the rational nature of the prohibition on homicide in Jewish law and the corrective role of the Noahide offence of bloodshed in Jewish criminal jurisprudence. Clearly, there are no rational grounds for treating the killing of a *terefah* as a less morally heinous act than indirect homicide. Indeed, the former might be considered to be worse, since it involves a direct act of murder, whereas the latter is indirect and, hence, less reprehensible from a moral point of view.[69] The principle of the preservation of society developed by Maimonides requires that this act be included in the Noahide offence of bloodshed. This, in turn, provides the basis for the invocation of divine sanctions upon an Israelite who kills a *terefah*. According to Maimonides's general theory of criminal jurisprudence outlined above, all forms of bloodshed are proscribed under Noahide law and, in principle at any rate, carry divine and extra-legal sanctions[70] in Jewish law.

The notion of a prohibition for which there is no concrete sanction is not foreign to the *halakhah*. It is widely used in the context of the Sabbath laws, where many acts are prohibited even though they carry no human sanction.[71] The analogy between the exemption of the killer of a *terefah* from capital punishment and the exemption of certain types of Sabbath-breakers from judicial penalties is stressed by R. Solomon Duran in a polemic work aimed at refuting non-Jewish criticisms of the *Talmud* and *halakhah*. R. Duran, a fifteenth-century Algerian authority, maintains that the term 'exempt' in relation to the killing of a *terefah* bears the same meaning as it does in relation to the laws of the Sabbath, i.e. 'exempt [from punishment] but [still] prohibited'.[72]

Another context in which the above theory is illuminating is the issue of grounds for prohibiting foeticide in the *halakhah*. Under Noahide law, foeticide is a capital crime.[73] It does not, however, carry any positive criminal sanction in Jewish law.[74] *Tosafot* cite the Talmudic principle: 'There is nothing permitted to an Israelite yet prohibited to a Noahide'[75] in order to prove that the *halakhah* does forbid unjustified foeticide to Israelites.[76] According to *Tosafot*, although Israelites 'are exempt [from capital punishment], it is not permitted'.[77] The centrality of *Tosafot's* formulation in the context of the *halakhah* on unjustified foeticide means that, in effect, the basis for this prohibition is derived from the general theory regarding the role of the Noahide system in Jewish criminal jurisprudence outlined above.[78]

It is noteworthy that Maimonides's attitude to abortion is a particularly stringent one. Even in relation to therapeutic abortion, Maimonides identifies the foetus as a pursuer threatening the life of the mother, in order to justify foeticide in such a case.[79] This justification is problematic since it ought equally to apply to a baby after birth, and it does not.[80] Moreover, the application of the pursuer principle to a foetus would appear to be specifically rejected in the *Talmud*.[81] The resolution of this difficulty in Maimonides's ruling has exercised many scholars, and the general consensus would appear to be on the lines that Maimonides found a certain strictness in relation to foeticide which required a stronger justification than the standard argument to the effect that a foetus is a non-person.[82] It is arguable, therefore, that the prohibition on foeticide in Noahide law does, in fact, constitute this strictness in relation to therapeutic abortion in Maimonides's ruling, even though he does not refer to it explicitly.

In terms of the general theory outlined above, the question of the sanctions to be imposed for unjustified foeticide in Jewish law is as important an issue as the establishment of a prohibition in the halakhic framework. Consequently, it is most significant that according to R. Meir Cohen, a prominent middle-eighteenth and early-nineteenth century commentator on the *Mishneh Torah*, the penalty for unjustified foeticide in Jewish law is death at the hands of Heaven.[83] R. Cohen's argument follows the theory exactly. After observing that foeticide is a capital crime in a Noahide code, R. Cohen concludes that it must also be prohibited in Jewish law. Since there is no positive sanction for unjustified foeticide, R. Cohen argues that any person guilty of unjustified foeticide is liable to death at the hands of Heaven. This view is also shared by other authorities.[84] It would appear, therefore, that the invocation of divine sanctions is one general response to marginal cases of bloodshed for which there are no positive penalties in Jewish criminal law.

The existence of a divine penalty in the case of killing a *terefah* is universally accepted and was reiterated in a recent *responsum* by R. Moses Feinstein on the question of dangerous medical treatment for the fatally ill. R. Feinstein sums up the position regarding the killing of a *terefah* in the *halakhah* as follows:

> The prohibition on killing a *terefah* applies equally to a Jew as to a Noahide by virtue of the Talmudic principle. 'There is nothing permitted to an Israelite yet forbidden to a Noahide.' Moreover, Maimonides explicitly provided that the killer of a *terefah* is exempt from human jurisdiction, implying that he is liable to Divine punishment in addition to having committed a transgression.[85]

R. Feinstein also observes that in the final analysis, Jews are always under a stricter obligation than Noahides, 'since they are sanctified by the commandments'.[86]

In the light of this analysis, it is clear that the fact that killing a *terefah* does not carry the death penalty in Jewish criminal law does not make it a permitted act. On the contrary, it constitutes a serious offence, namely bloodshed, and it also carries a divine sanction. Now, it is obvious that in the context of a modern, secular, pluralistic society, divine sanctions hardly constitute significant deterrents, except for a small minority of religious people. The major conclusion to be drawn from this sanction in Jewish law is, therefore, that those involved in the killing of the fatally ill ought not to be subject to the same penalties as the murderers of viable individuals.

Extra-Legal Penalties for the Offence of Bloodshed in Jewish Law

Immediately subsequent to the provisions regarding indirect killing and suicide cited above, Maimonides states as follows:

Regarding any of these or similar murderers who are not subject to being condemned to die by verdict of the court, if a king of Israel wishes to put them to death by royal decree and for the sake of improving society, he has a right to do so. Similarly, if the court deems it proper to put them to death as an emergency measure, it has the authority to do so as it deems fit, provided that the circumstances would warrant such action.[87]

Moreover, even if circumstances are such that the needs of the time do not demand the deaths of the killers concerned, it is nevertheless the duty of the court to take the following action against them:

to flog them almost to the point of death, to imprison them in a fortress or a prison for many years, and to inflict severe punishment on them in order to frighten and terrify other wicked persons, lest such a case become a pitfall and a snare, enticing one to say, 'I will arrange to kill my enemy in a roundabout way as did so-and-so, and then I will be acquitted.'[88]

Maimonides's specification of these extra-legal penalties is undoubtedly motivated by the general theory outlined above, according to which bloodshed is the ultimate threat to civilised society and cannot, therefore, be allowed to go unpunished. In this respect, it is noteworthy that the extra-legal jurisdiction of the king and court extends to all those killers guilty of bloodshed for whom there is no capital punishment, and not only to indirect killers and suicides. The wide scope of this provision is implicit in Maimonides's use of the phrase, 'or similar murderers' in the first of the above quotations. Clearly, the killer of a *terefah* falls into this category and, in addition to divine punishment, is also subject to the extra-legal jurisdiction of the king and court.[89]

Now, the authority of the court to impose extra-legal sanctions in order to protect religious and moral standards is well established in the *halakhah*.[90] The authority of the king, however, is not so clear.[91] Although the king is entitled to execute those who rebel against him,[92] there is no clear source for his authority to punish killers who are exempt from regular criminal sanctions. The question arises, therefore, as to the basis for Maimonides's ruling that the king has the right to put to death such murderers for the sake of improving society.

Before proceeding to an integrated theoretical solution to this problem, it is noteworthy that Maimonides makes a similar point with regard to the role of the king in relation to another class of criminals who are not subject to the regular penalties of the criminal law. In the following extract, Maimonides refers to those exempt from capital punishment as a result of insufficient or technically defective evidence, or lack of a formal warning:

> If a person kills another and there is no clear evidence, or if no warning has been given him, or there is only one witness, or if one kills accidentally a person whom he hated, the king may, if the exigency of the hour demands it, put him to death in order to ensure the stability of the social order. He may put to death many offenders in one day, hang them, and suffer them to be hanging for a long time so as to put fear in the hearts of others and break the power of the wicked.[93]

The salient feature of all the cases mentioned in this provision is that they constitute culpable forms of bloodshed in the Noahide laws. Under these laws, the murderer does not require a warning, and may be executed on the testimony of one witness alone.[94] The king is therefore empowered, at least according to Maimonides, to put criminals to death on the basis of evidence which would only be acceptable under the Noahide code.

The basis of Maimonides's views concerning the extra-legal jurisdiction of the king in relation to murderers who fall outside the jurisdiction of the regular human court would now appear to be clear. The king is authorised to enforce the provisions of the Noahide prohibition on bloodshed, since the enforcement of this prohibition is a necessary prerequisite for the preservation of society, and the king is entrusted with the general welfare of the people over whom he rules.[95] The link between the king's jurisdiction in this area and the Noahide code is in fact suggested by R. Meir Cohen, whose views on divine sanctions for foeticide in Jewish law were cited above. According to R. Cohen: ' . . . an Israelite king is authorised by virtue of his role as the preserver of the social order to act according to the general Noahide code, and this is a rational principle'.[96] R. Cohen identifies the king's general role in preserving society with the enforcement of the Noahide laws. He also emphasises the rational nature of this link. According to this view, therefore, Maimonides is merely giving his theory of the role of the Noahide offence of bloodshed in Jewish criminal jurisprudence outlined in the previous section a practical, institutional form. In his capacity as monarch the king is entrusted with the maintenance of civilised society, and since bloodshed constitutes the most basic threat to such a society he must take all the necessary steps to ensure its eradication.

The question that arises is the extent to which Noahide laws other than bloodshed also fall into this category. Although Maimonides regards bloodshed as the most serious threat to society, there would appear to be some grounds for arguing that Noahide offences such as sexual licentiousness and theft are equally dangerous.[97] Indeed, the view that the king's jurisdiction applies to the whole range of Noahide offences is expressed in halakhic literature.[98] According to R. Meir Plotzki, the king's jurisdiction would also apply to offences involving sexual licentiousness and any crime against the 'natural order' of society.[99] There would also appear to be some grounds for extending this jurisdiction to theft, which is also forbidden under the Noahide laws.[100] It is arguable, therefore, at least from a theoretical point of view, that the king's extra-legal jurisdiction might apply to the whole Noahide code, and not merely to the offence of bloodshed.

Another issue that presents itself for discussion in this context is the relationship between the extra-legal jurisdiction of the king and that of the court. Both institutions enjoy extra-legal jurisdiction with respect to killers exempt from capital punishment. The king's jurisdiction would, however, appear to be somewhat wider than that of the court.[101] It has already been observed that the court may only mete out extra-legal penalties as an 'emergency measure' and in order to 'safeguard a cause'.[102] Moreover, with regard to killing those against whom there is defective evidence or lack of a formal warning, Maimonides specifies the king, rather than the court, as the relevant punitive agency.[103] Clearly, extra-legal procedures on the part of the court must be restricted to the minimum, for otherwise the whole structure of the legal system would be threatened. Any departure from the rules of evidence by a court is bound to detract from the authority of the system as a whole. Consequently, the king, rather than the court, ought to be empowered to remedy the breach in public morality by executing those against whom the evidence is inconclusive or defective. The king's jurisdiction may, therefore, be of a more general nature than that of the court, which is still subject, albeit in a somewhat flexible fashion, to the strictly legal forms of the *halakhah*.[104]

A distinction along these lines is made by R. Plotzki, who differentiates between the 'natural' order of the Noahide laws and the order of the Torah.[105] The former is free from all formal constraints such as evidence, and the restrictive scope of various offences. The latter, on the other hand, is limited in both form and content. This difference reflects different stages in the religious and moral state of society. Citing the opinion of R. Nissim referred to above, R. Plotzki observes that Jewish criminal law is applicable only to a society operating at a high religious and spiritual level. Once Jewish society falls below this level, the king's jurisdiction alone is applicable, until such time as the former standard is regained.[106] At the lower level of social development, there is no justification for the restrictions on the administration of capital punishment imposed by the *halakhah.* The rational basis for the enforcement of the Noahide prohibition on bloodshed is sufficient to justify the stringent punishment of all offenders.[107] Only at the higher stages of religious and moral development are the procedural and evidentiary requirements of Jewish criminal law justified.

In the light of this view of the role of the king and court in relation to the murder of a *terefah,* it is arguable that cases involving the killing of the fatally ill ought to be dealt with in an extra-legal fashion by bodies operating on the basis of fairly flexible principles of both procedure and punishment. The fact that the sources cited above only deal with the court and the king does not constitute a serious objection to the application of the principles contained therein to contemporary times, since there is a well-established view in Rabbinic literature that these ancient institutions have had their parallels in Jewish communal institutions throughout the ages. This is especially true of institutions arising in the State of Israel.[108] It may, therefore, be concluded that according to Jewish law the punishment meted out to those involved in the killing of a fatally ill patient is a matter of pure discretion and ought not to be dealt with in the same way as regular homicide in the criminal courts.[109] The difference between this approach and that of many other systems is that in Jewish law, the exemption of the killer of a fatally ill person is explicit, whereas in other systems it is implicit, i.e. it depends upon an executive or legislative act of pardon.[110] This difference was noted by R. Solomon Duran, whose polemic in defence of Talmudic law was mentioned above.[111] According to R. Duran, the *ab initio* exclusion of the crime of murdering a *terefah* from human jurisdiction is preferable to the course adopted in non-

Jewish law, in which the death sentence in this type of case is mitigated by a royal pardon. R. Duran argues that the latter approach obscures the true grounds for not administering capital punishment, and leaves the public believing that justice was simply not done. The halakhic approach is preferable since it excludes the death penalty in this type of case from the very outset and does not, therefore, prejudice the public perception of justice in the law as does the approach based upon royal pardon. Irrespective of the merits of R. Duran's claim in the context of comparative jurisprudence,[112] his point that the *halakhah* excludes the murder of a *terefah* from the jurisdiction of the regular criminal court supports the line of argument in this section. Both the procedure and the penalties for those involved in the killing of the fatally ill ought to rest in the hands of bodies outside the regular court system. These bodies would operate on the basis of discretionary principles, the most significant of which is the moral condition of society. Such bodies would possess wide punitive powers, including that of capital punishment.

In the course of this chapter, it has been demonstrated that, in Maimonides's view at least, the exemption of the killer of a *terefah* from capital punishment is of marginal significance only, since the *halakhah* treats such a killing as an offence and makes the perpetrator liable to both divine and human penalties. Now, it has already been observed that although unjustified foeticide carries no specified sanction in Jewish criminal law, it is prohibited and does carry a similar range of penalties. In the case of justified abortion—where the mother's life is jeopardised by the continuation of the pregnancy—foeticide is permitted since, according to most authorities, a foetus is not considered a living being.[113] Is there any provision in halakhic literature for drawing a similar distinction with regard to the *terefah,* i.e. does the fatal nature of his disease provide a basis for arguing that in a situation of conflict between two lives the viable life should be preferred to the non-viable? This question and its ramifications for the principle of the value of human life in Jewish law will be discussed in the course of the following two chapters.

Notes
1. See *M. Hull.* 3:1; *Hull.* 42a; Maimonides, *Hil. Shehitah* 10-9; *Shulhan Arukh, Yoreh Deah, Hil. Terefot.*

2. *Hull.* 54a. This point is expressed most forcefully in the following extract from Maimonides, *Hil. Shehitah* 10:12–13:

> One may not under any circumstances add to this list of causes of *terefah*, for in the case of any other defect in an animal, beast or bird, beyond those which the Sages of former generations have enumerated, and to which the contemporary Israelite courts of law have given their assent, it is possible for the animal to go on living, even if our own medical knowledge assures us that it cannot eventually survive. Conversely, as regards the defects which the Sages have enumerated, concerning which they have said that they render the animal *terefah*, even if it should appear from our present knowledge of medicine that some of them are not fatal and that the animal can survive them, one must go only by what the Sages have enumerated as it is said, 'According to the law which they shall teach you' [*Deut.* 7:11].

3. *Hull.* 58a; Maimonides, *Hil, Shehitah* 11:1; *Tur, Yoreh Deah* 57; *Shulhan Arukh, Yoreh Deah* 57:18.

4. *Tur. id.; Shulhan Arukh, id.; Siftei Kohen, Shulhan Arukh* 57:48.

5. *Yad Remah, Sanh.* 78a. *s.v. amar Rava; Minhat Hinukh* no.34.

6. *Hil. Rozeah* 2:8.

7. See *Resp. Iggrot Moshe, Yoreh Deah* 3 no. 37 and *Hoshen Mishpat* 2 no. 73; R. Moses Hirschler, 'The obligation to save life' (Heb.), *Halakhah Urefuah* 2 (5741) 49. The view expressed by A. Steinberg to the effect that Rashi restricts the human *terefah* to those symptoms specified in relation to animals would appear to be too simplistic ('Mercy-Killing in the light of the *Halakhah'* (Heb.), *Sefer Assia,* ed. A. Steinberg (Jerusalem, 5743). Although Rashi provides two illustrations from the list of specified animal *terefot* in his commentary on *Sanhedrin* 78a *s.v. hakol modim,* the subject of which is the human *terefah*, there is little doubt that his intention is merely to illustrate the condition and not to provide an exhaustive definition of it.

8. *Resp. Iggrot Moshe, Hoshen Mishpat* 2 no. 73:4.

9. *Resp. Ahiezer, Yoreh Deah* no. 16:6; Hirshler, *op. cit.* p.49. Note that according to R. Grodzinski, human *tarfut* applies to a disease, and not only to external wounds, cf. R. Immanuel Jacobovitz, 'Concerning the possibility of permitting the precipitation of the death of a fatally ill patient in severe pain' (Heb.), *Hapardes* 31 (5717) 43.

10. For the categorisation of cancer as a form of human *tarfut,* see R. Elijah Katz, 'Regarding the issue of disconnecting a fatally ill patient from a respirator' (Heb.), *Tehumin* 3 (5741) 297.

11. *Yeb.* 120b–121a; Maimonides, *Hil. Gerushin* 13:16–18; *Tur, Even Haezer* 17; *Shulhan Arukh, Even Haezer* 17:30–2.

12. *M. Yeb.* 16:4; Ramban, *Yeb.* 120b *s.v. umi matsit;* Rashba, *Yeb.* 120 *s.v.umi matsit; Maggid Mishneh, Hil. Gerushin* 13:16 *s.v. vekakh nireh; Kesef Mishneh, Hil. Gerushin* 13:16 *s.v. vekhen im; Tur, id.; Shulhan Arukh, ibid.* 32. Also see *Resp. Mishpetei Uziel, Even Haezer* no. 79; *Resp. Ziz Eliezer* 1 no. 23.

13. *Tosafot Gitt.* 57b *s.v. venikar bemokho; Tosafot Erub.* 7a *s.v. kegaon shidra; Kesef Mishneh, id.; Tosafot Yom Tov, M. Yeb.* 16:4.

14. The issue here is the possibility of placing an absolute time limit on a human *terefah's* life-span. All authorities agree that a *terefah* cannot

survive for much longer than a year: see R. Saul Nathanson, *Divrei Saul, Yoreh Deah, Hil. Avelut* 394:3.

15. *Yad Remah, Sanh.* 78a, *s.v. amar Raba; Shittah Mekubetset, B.K.* 26a, *s.v. vekhatav harav Yosef Halevi ibn Migash; Minhat Hinukh* no. 34; H. Cohn, 'On the dichotomy of divinity and humanity in Jewish law', in *Euthanasia,* ed. A. Carmi (Berlin, 1984), p.38.

16. *Resp. Ginat Veradim* 2, *Even Haezer* n.2:4.

17. *Resp. Maggid Mereshit* no. 2 (9a). The argument here is that where the wife is a *terefah,* her status as a 'dead person' means that her husband is not marrying her sister 'in her lifetime', *Lev.* 18:18.

18. *Resp. Hikrei Lev, Even Haezer* no. 11; *Petah Hadevir* 2 *Orah Hayyim,* 199; *Petah Hadevir* 4 *Orah Hayyim,* 229; *Resp. Mishpetei Uziel, Even Haezer* no. 79; *Resp. Yabia Omer* 4, *Even Haezer* no. 1:4. A detailed account of all the legal material relating to the status of a *terefah* is clearly beyond the scope of this book, and the outline in the body of the text is sufficient for the purpose of indicating the underlying concept of human *tarfut* in Jewish law.

19. See above, notes 28, 59.

20. See above, n.53.

21. See *Resp. Iggrot Moshe, Hoshen Mishpat* 2 no. 73.

22. See p.9.

23. See p.10.

24. *Sanh.* 78a.

25. Maimonides, *Hil. Rozeah* 2:8. On the burden of proof, see Cohn, *op. cit.* p.57. The centrality of Maimonides's formulation of this *halakhah* in any discussion of the killing of a *terefah* in Jewish law is due to the unique scope of his code, which is the only such work to embrace this aspect of the criminal law. For a discussion of the unique scope of Maimonides's Code, see I. Twersky, *Introduction to the Code of Maimonides* (New Haven, 1980), ch. 3. On the legal significance of the innovative approach adopted by Maimonides to the process of the codification of Jewish law, see M. Elon, *Hamishpat Haivri* (Jerusalem, 5737), 980.

26. *Sanh.* 78a.

27. See n.15 above.

28. *Sanh.* 78a; Maimonides, *Hil. Rozeah* 2:7.

29. *Kidd.* 43a. It is noteworthy that in the course of the discussion, the *Talmud* suggests that divine punishment would be a universally acceptable sanction in such a case.

30. *Sanh.* 77a.

31. *B.K.* 91b. The obvious question of the impracticality of punishing a suicide is answered in terms of eternal, rather than terrestial life, i.e. the individual concerned is deprived of his share in the 'world-to-come'; see *Sem.* 2:1 and *Torah Temimah, Gen.* ch. 9, no. 8.

32. In the case of the assassin and the slave, the principal is not liable since there is no 'offence by proxy' in Jewish law *(Kidd.* 43a). Binding a person before a wild beast does not carry the death penalty if the individual concerned is killed, since the act is still too indirect in nature *(Sanh.* 77a). Capital punishment is excluded in the case of a suicide for obvious reasons: see n.31 above.

33. Maimonides, *Hil. Rozeah* 2:2–3.

34. *Gen. Rabbah* 34:14.

35. There are seven basic Noahide laws, i.e. the offences of idolatry, blasphemy, bloodshed, forbidden sexual relations, theft, tearing a

limb from a living animal, and the positive obligation to set up a
system of justice: see *T.A. Zar.* 8:4; *Sanh.* 67a; Maimonides, *Hil,
Melakhim* 9:1. According to Rabbinic tradition, six of these laws
were given to Adam, whilst the seventh, (the prohibition on tearing a
limb from a living creature) was given to Noah. The title 'Noahide
laws' is, therefore, derived from the seventh law, given to Noah and
his descendants. Each of these seven laws is subdivided into further
offences which generally extend beyond the scope of halakhic
provisions in the same area. This is particularly evident in the case
of bloodshed, which covers many offences not incorporated into the
halakhic category of homicide: see *Encyclopaedia Talmudit* 3, p.351.
For a general survey of the legal significance of these laws, see S.
Berman, 'Noahide laws', in *The Principles of Jewish Law,* ed. M.
Elon (Jerusalem, 1975) 708. There is a considerable body of opinion
to the effect that the Noahide laws constitute a Natural law
dimension in the *halakhah,* i.e. they are binding by virtue of reason
rather than revelation. This theory is generally based upon
Maimonidean texts and, in particular, *Hil. Melakhim* 9:11: see S.
Atlas, *Netivim Bemishpat Ivri* (New York 5738) p.17; D. Novak, *The
Image of the Non-Jew in Judaism* (New York, 1983) 290; N. Lamm
and A. Kirschenbaum, 'Freedom and constraint in the Jewish
judicial process', *Cardozo Law Review* (1970), 110. The opposite
view is taken by M. Fox, 'Maimonides and Aquinas on Natural law',
Dine Israel 5 (1972), 1; J. Faur, *Iyunim Bemishnah Torah: Sefer
Hamada* (Jerusalem, 5738), 151 and this debate is referred to below
at notes 61-68. Although the general issue of the Noahide laws as a
Natural law system is clearly beyond the scope of this book, it might
be useful to observe that whilst it is unlikely that the *halakhah*
recognises the notion of a higher law than itself, it may nevertheless
accept a weaker version of the Natural law doctrine according to
which there are certain rules which must be present in a legal system
in order to ensure the viability of any civilised society: see H. Hart,
The Concept of Law (Oxford, 1964), ch. 9; J. Harris, *Legal
Philosophies* (London, 1980), ch. 2; and n.60 below. This indeed is
the approach which will be developed in the course of the present
chapter, since much of the argument in the body of the text turns on
the notion that the offence of bloodshed in the Noahide code
constitutes a minimum standard, below which the legal system of
any civilised society, including a Jewish one, cannot afford to
fall.

36. *Gen. Rabbah* 34:14; Maimonides, *Hil. Melakhim* 9:4.
37. The nature of the relationship between Noahide law and the
    provisions of the *halakhah* is a complex topic: see *Shab.* 135a; *Sanh.*
    59a; *Resp. Rashbash* no. 543; *Bet Haotsar* 1, Principle 1, sec. 7;
    M. Potolsky, 'The Rabbinic rule "No rules are derived from before
    Sinai"' (Heb.), *Dine Israel* 6 (5736), 195. In the context of the present
    chapter, the relationship between the Noahide offence of bloodshed
    and the *halakhah* will be examined in detail. It would, however,
    appear to be arguable, at least on prima-facie grounds, that an
    offence such as the one under consideration ought not to be
    controlled by the Noahide prohibition since the *halakhah* specifically
    excludes the perpetrator from human law: see R. Zvi Hayyes,

Torat Neviim, ch. 11 in *Kol Kitvei Marats Hayyes* 1 (Jerusalem, 5718), 71 for an argument on similar lines. Also see Potolsky, *ibid.,* 208.

38. *Sanh.* 57a; *Gen. Rabbah* 34:14; Maimonides, *Hil. Melakhim* 9:4.

39. *Midrash Halakhah* on the Book of *Exodus.* The *Mekhilta* is a Tannaitic production comprising a collection of *braitot.* On the legal significance of these *Midrashim,* see Elon, *op. cit.* p.243.

40. *Ex.* 21:14: 'And if a man come presumptuously upon his neighbour, to slay him with guile, from off My altar you shall take him, that he may die.' The implication here is that only the murder of a 'neighbour' i.e. fellow Israelite, carries the death penalty.

41. *Mekhilta Derabbi Yishmael, Masekhta D'Nezikin,* 4, ed. H. Horowitz, I. Rabin, 263.

42. *Sanh.* 59a; see *Tosafot, Sanh.* 59a *s.v. mi ika; Tosafot, Hull.* 33a *s.v. ehad oved kokhavim* and n.77 below.

43. *Derashot Haran* no. 11, cf. R. Issac Abrabanel's *Commentary on the Torah, Deut.* 17, sec. 4. R. Nissim cites *A. Zar.* 8b in support of this contention. According to that source, 'when the Sanhedrin saw that murderers were so prevalent that they could not be properly dealt with judicially, they said: Rather let us be exiled from place to place than pronounce them guilty . . . '. On the basis of this dictum, R. Nissim concludes that Jewish criminal law is suspended as long as the Noahide offence of bloodshed is not generally enforced.

44. See H. Cohn, 'Divine punishment', in *The Principles of Jewish Law, op. cit.,* p.522, and 'The secularization of divine law', in *Jewish Law in Ancient and Modern Israel,* ed. H. Cohn (New York, 1971), p.12ff.; B. Jackson, *Essays in Jewish and Comparative Legal History* (Leiden, 1975), pp.54, 265. The notion of divine retribution may be regarded as one of the central religious features of Jewish law: see B. Jackson, 'The concept of religious law in Judaism', *Aufsteig und Niedergang der Romischen Welt* 19 (1979), 33. On the halakhic concept of divine jurisdiction *(dinei shamayim)* see Elon, *op. cit.* p.172; S. Federbusch, *Hamussar Vehamishpat Beyisrael* (Jerusalem, 5739), p.140; and *Encyclopaedia Talmudit* 7, p.382.

45. This expression indicates that even indirect homicide is forbidden, which further supports the thesis advanced in the main body of the text regarding the liability of Israelites to all the provisions of the Noahide prohibition on bloodshed. Indeed, this is the position adopted by various authorities: see *Resp. Temim Deim* no. 203; *Bah, Yoreh Deah* 158; cf. *Taz, Yoreh Deah* 158:1.

46. Maimonides, *Hil. Rozeah* 4:11. In *Hil. Avodah Zarah* 11:1, Maimonides extends this ruling to idolators.

47. *Kesef Mishneh, Hil. Rozeah* 2:11; Ravan, *B.K.* 113a, *Yereim Hashalem,* 175.

48. See Novak, *op. cit.,* p.171.

49. See above n.36.

50. There is no indication in *Gen. Rabbah* 34:13 that these offences carry any penalty of a divine nature. In their critical edition of the *Midrash,* J. Theodor and H. Albeck *(Gen. Rabbah,* 324 n.8) observe that under the influence of Maimonides's ruling, editions of the *Midrash* provided that the offenders in such cases were indeed liable to divine sanctions. Divine punishment for inflicting minor injuries upon oneself is, in fact, mentioned in the Leiden manuscripts

of the *Tosefta, B.K.* 9; see R. Menaham Kasher, *Torah Shelemah* 2 (New York 5711), *Gen.* 9 no. 27. There is, however, no extant source providing divine punishment in cases of indirect killing or suicide.

51. *Kesef Mishneh, Hil. Rozeah* 2:2.

52. *Kidd.* 43a.

53. *Hil. Melakhim* 9:4.

54. See *Gen. Rabbah* 34:14. As yet, no textual variation incorporating the killing of a *terefah* into this *Midrash* has come to light.

55. *Mekorei Harambam Lerashash, Hil. Melakhim* 9:4; *Or Sameah, Hil. Rozeah* 4:3; *Mirkevet Hamishneh, Hil. Melakhim* 9:4; *Maaseh Rokeah, Hil. Melakhim* 9:4.

56. See n.35.

57. *Hil. Melakhim* 9:1. See *Atlas, op. cit.,* p.17. The inclination of the reason may not be strong enough to provide the basis for a binding law, i.e. the 'determination of reason' mentioned in *Hil. Melakhim* 8:11. Nevertheless, it is sufficiently strong to establish the rational character of these laws.

58. *Hil. Melakhim* 8:11, cf. *Mishnat Rabbi Eliezer,* ed. H. Enelow (New York, 1933) 121, according to which the 'pious of the nations of the world' are only those who perform the Noahide laws 'because our father Noah commanded us by the mouth of God . . . But if they fulfil the Seven Commandments [of the Noahide Code] . . . of their own accord for so does reason determine . . . they receive their reward only in this world.' However, it is not clear that his *Midrash* constitutes a source for Maimonides's ruling. For various suggestions with regard to such a source, see *Resp. Rashbash* no. 543; *Or Sameah, Hil Issurei Biah,* 3:2. According to Novak, *op. cit.,* p.288, the source of this ruling lies in Maimonides's distinction between wisdom and spiritual perfection.

59. J. Katz, *Exclusiveness and Tolerance* (New York, 1962) 175; Schwartzchild, *op. cit.* p.301; Fox, *op. cit.,* p.14; Faur, *op. cit.,* p.151, n.43; Lamm and Kirschenbaum, *op. cit.,* p.117. This reading is also found in *Resp. Maharam Alashkar* no. 117 and is supported by R. Abraham Kook, *Iggrot Rayah* (Jerusalem, 5721) 1 no. 99.

60. *Hil. Melakhim* 10:11.

61. See n.35. The issue of the rational basis of the Noahide system as a whole is an important one in the debate as to whether or not this system is a Natural law system. It has also been observed that there is a weaker version of the Natural law doctrine typified by Hart's notion of the 'minimum content of Natural law' which might be more apposite in the context of the *halakhah.* According to Hart:

> Reflections on some very obvious generalisations—indeed truisms—concerning human nature and the world in which men live, show that as long as these hold good, there are certain rules of conduct which any social organisation must contain if it is to be viable. Such rules do, in fact, constitute a common element in the law and conventional morality of all societies which have progressed to the point where these are distinguished as different forms of social control. With them are found, both in law and morals, much that is peculiar to a particular society and much that may be seen as arbitrary or a matter of choice. Such universally recognised principles

> of conduct which have a basis in elementary truths concerning
> human beings, their natural environment and aims, may be
> considered the minimum content of Natural law *[Concept of
> Law,* Oxford, 1964 p.188].

Clearly, bloodshed is a fundamental element in the notion of the
'minimum content of Natural law' presented in this passage, and, as will
be shown in the course of this section, the strong emphasis on the rational
nature of the prohibition on all forms of homicide in halakhic sources in
general, and Maimonides's *Mishneh Torah* in particular, would seem to
support the contention that this notion is an illuminating one in the
context of Jewish law. For further discussion of this point, see n.50.

62. *Sanh.* 74a. On the question of whether non-Jews are liable to suffer
    martyrdom in similar circumstances, see *Mishneh Lemelekh, Hil.,
    Melakhim* 10:2; *Resp. Koah Shor* no.2; *Minhat Hinukh* no.296 in
    which it is answered in the affirmative. Also see Faur, op. cit. p.161.

63. See Faur, *id.* On the legal status of rational principles *(sevarah)* in
    the *halakhah,* see Elon, *op. cit.,* pp.2, 805.

64. *Sanh.* 74a. An analogy is drawn between the two crimes on the basis
    of their juxtaposition in Scripture *(Deut.* 22:26): see Elon, op. cit.
    pp.290, 808.

65. *M. Sanh.* 9:5; *Sanh.* 81b; Maimonides, *Hil. Rozeah* 4:8.

66. This phrase is similar to the one used by Maimonides in relation to
    the enforcement of the whole of the Noahide code: see *Hil.
    Melakhim* 10:11. It also provides further support for the contention
    that Hart's notion of the 'minimum content of Natural law' is an
    illuminating one in the context of the prohibition on all forms of
    bloodshed in Jewish law (n. 61 above). In this respect, it is
    noteworthy that the one prominent medieval Jewish thinker who
    does actually deal with Natural law does so only in the context of
    murder, robbery, or theft. He also presents it in terms of the
    preservation of society. According to R. Joseph Albo:

    > The purpose of Natural law is to repress wrong and to
    > promote right in order that people be kept away from theft,
    > robbery and murder, that society may be able to exist among
    > men and everyone be safe from the wrongdoer and the
    > oppressor *[Sefer Ikkarim* 1:7].

    Albo's concept of Natural law doctrine is discussed by R. Lerner,
    'Natural Law in Albo's Book of Roots', in *Ancients and Moderns,* ed.
    J. Crospey (New York, 1964), p.132, and the conclusion reached is
    that his doctrine is more properly referred to as a 'quasi-Natural
    law'. This would appear once again to correspond closely to Hart's
    notion of the minimum content of Natural law, the origin of which is
    usually traced to Thomas Hobbes's *(Leviathan,* ch. 13). In addition
    to homicide, it is arguable that the Noahide prohibitions on theft
    and forbidden sexual relations also constitute elements in this
    minimum content of Natural law in the *halakhah.* Albo's language
    would certainly indicate that this was the case with regard to theft.
    Support for the rational basis of the laws against licentiousness may
    be derived from the fact that the king may very well be empowered
    to impose extra-judicial sanctions upon those who infringe them:
    see p. 33. There is, however, little certainty regarding this point, and
    at this stage, it would probably be best to confine the scope of even
    this minimum Natural law doctrine in *halakhah* to the area of
    bloodshed alone, cf. notes 97, 98.

67. Maimonides, *Hil. Rozeah* 4:9.
68. *Hil. Melakhim* 10:11. It is significant that this term is employed in relation to the enforcement of the Noahide code. Non-enforcement would clearly lead to the breakdown of society. This argument is typically used with respect to the weaker form of the Natural law doctrine referred to in notes 61 and 66 above. In the context of punishment, it is noteworthy that criminal procedure for Noahides is much stricter than in the case of Israelites: see *Sanh.* 57b and I. Weiss, *Dor Dor Vedorshav* (Berlin, 1923), p.158. Presumably, the rational character of the Noahide code is the underlying reason for the absence of strict rules of criminal procedure: see R. Elihah Benamozegh, *Israel et L'Humanite* (Paris, 1914), p.688; Atlas, *op. cit.* p.2. According to Novak, *op. cit.,* p. 179, the apparently unfair disparity between Noahide and Jewish law in this area can be explained in historical terms, i.e. Jewish reverence for human life was greater than that of the Roman Empire. Hence, Jewish law was far more cautious in its willingness to require capital punishment than were the Romans, who used frequent executions as a method of political terror.
69. The distinction between direct acts and indirect acts in terms of moral culpability is widely accepted in both law and morality. For a discussion of this distinction in relation to the termination of the lives of the critically ill, see p.72.
70. See p.31 below.
71. See *Shab.* 3a; *Shab.* 107a; Maimonides, *Hil. Shabbat* 1:3.
72. *Milkhemet Mitzva* 32b *s.v. od heshiv,* and see p.35 for R. Duran's comparison between Jewish and Gentile law on this point.
73. *Sanh.* 57b, cf. *Gen. Rabbah* 34:13. See Weiss, *op. cit.* p.23; V. Aptowitzer, 'The status of the embryo in Jewish law', *Jewish Quarterly Review* ns 15 (1924), 113; G. Alon, *Mehkarim Betoldot Yisrael* (Tel Aviv, 5727), p.280 for a historical approach to the apparent discrepancy between Noahide and Jewish law in this area. The details of the Noahide prohibition are summarised in the following: R. David Bleich, *Contemporary Halakhic Problems* 1 (New York 1977), p.367; R. Michel Stern, *Harefuah Leor Hahalakhah* (Jerusalem, 5740) pt. 1, sec. 3. Also see Novak, *op. cit.,* p.185.
74. Rashi, *Sanh.* 72b *s.v. yatza;* Yad Remah, *Sanh.* 57a 72b; Meiri, *Sanh.* 72b; Ramban, *Torat Haadam* in *Kol Kitvei Haramban* (Jerusalem, 5724) 29; M. Weinfeld, 'The genuine Jewish attitude towards abortion' (Heb.), *Zion* 42 (5737), 130; Bleich, *ibid.,* 326; Stern, *ibid.,* pt 1, sec. 1, chs. 1–4. A person who causes a woman to miscarry is, however, obliged to compensate her husband for the loss of the foetus: *Ex.* 21:22; *Arak.* 7a; *Resp. Ziz Eliezer* 9 no. 51:3.
75. *Sanh.* 59a. The scope of this rule regarding foeticide in the framework of Jewish law is debated in recent literature: see *Resp. Ziz Eliezer* 9 no. 51:3:1; Potolsky, *op. cit.* p.215; R. Erusi, 'Abortion—theory and practice in the *halakhah*' (Heb.), *Dine Israel* 8 (5737), 125. That it is an important feature of the halakhic attitude towards unjustified foeticide is, however, beyond any doubt.
76. Therapeutic abortion is permitted in Jewish law: *M. Ohol.* 7:6; Maimonides, *Hil. Rozeah* 1:9; *Shulhan Arukh, Hoshen Mishpat* 452:2. The scope of this permission is, however, a matter of extensive debate amongst halakhic authorities: see Bleich, *op. cit.,*

p.347; Stern, *op. cit.*, pt 1, sec. 2. In particular, note the recent debate concerning the permissibility of aborting a foetus suffering from Tay-Sachs disease: *Resp. Ziz Eliezer* 13 no. 102; R. Moses Feinstein, 'On the law concerning the killing of a foetus' (Heb.), in *R. Ezekiel Abramski Memorial Volume*, ed. M. Hirschler (Jerusalem, 5735), 462; *Resp. Ziz Eliezer* 14 no. 78.

77. *Tosafot, Sanh.* 59a *s.v. mi ika; Hull.* 33a *s.v. ehad oved kokhavim.*
78. See Novak, *op. cit.* p.185; Stern, *op. cit.*, pt 1, sec. 1, ch. 7.
79. Maimonides, *Hil. Rozeah* 1:9.
80. Maimonides, *id.*
81. *Sanh.* 72b.
82. See *Resp. Noda Beyehuda* 2, *Hoshen Mishpat* no. 59; *Resp. Havot Yair* no. 31; *Resp. Koah Shor* no. 20; *Hiddushei Rabbi Hayyim Halevi, Hil. Rozeah* 1:9; Bleich, *op. cit.* p.348; Stern, *op. cit.*, pt 1, sec. 1, ch. 8.
83. *Or Sameah, Hil. Issurei Biah* 3:2; *Meshekh Hokhmah, Parashat Vayakhel s.v. shabbat shabbaton.* Also note the words of R. Menahem Meiri *(Sanh.* 57b) to the effect that Noahides are liable to capital punishment for acts of bloodshed for which Israelites go unpunished. The reason for this is 'since even in the case of Israelites, the king can punish them'. As the offences for which a Noahide is subject to the death penalty include foeticide, it might be argued that according to R. Meiri, such an act would fall under the special jurisdiction of the king outlined in the following section: see below n.93.
84. See Bleich, *op. cit.*, p.331; Stern, *op. cit.*, pt 1, sec. 1, ch. 13.
85. *Resp. Iggrot Moshe, Yoreh Deah* no. 36.
86. *Id.*
87. Maimonides, *Hil. Rozeah* 2:4.
88. Maimonides, *Hil. Rozeah* 2:5.
89. Also see *Hil. Rozeah* 1:13, 2:7, 2:11 and 3:10–11 for other instances in which Maimonides implies that the killers in question, although exempt from human jurisdiction are nevertheless liable to penalties of an extra-legal nature.
90. The two categories most commonly referred to in this context are those of 'emergency measures' *(hora'at sha'ah)* and 'safeguarding a cause' *(midgar milta):* see *Yeb.* 90b; Maimonides, *Hil. Mamrim* 2:4; Elon, *op. cit.* pp.2, 421; R. Jacob Ginzburg, *Mishpatim Leyisrael* (Jerusalem, 5716), ch. 4; E. Quint and N. Hecht, *Jewish Jurisprudence,* (New York, 1980), ch. 2.
91. In general, the king is excluded from any judicial, and presumably, extra-judical role: see *M. Sanh.* 2:2; *Sanh.* 18b; Maimonides, *Hil. Sanhedrin* 2:4–5. For a detailed study of the judicial role of the king of Israel, see J. Blidstein, *Ikkronot Mediniim Bemishnat Harambam* (Bar-Ilan, 5743), ch. 5.
92. *Sanh.* 49a; Maimonides, *Hil Melakhim* 3:8.
93. Maimonides, *Hil. Melakhim* 3:10. For the background to the permission to leave offenders hanging for a long time in contravention of the biblical prohibition in *Deut.* 21:23, see *T. Sanh.* 21:10; *Yeb.* 79a; Ramban, *Deut.* 21:22; *Resp. Hatam Sofer, Orah Hayyim* no. 208. In the *Guide for the Perplexed* 3:40, Maimonides makes a general reference to the power of the king to punish murderers who, for some reason or another, escape the death penalty: 'If the court of

justice cannot sentence him to death, the king may find him guilty
who has the power to sentence to death on circumstantial evidence.'
Also see *Encyclopaedia Talmudit* 5, p.233, n.31.

94. *Gen. Rabbah* 34-14; *Sanh.* 57a; Maimonides, *Hil. Melakhim* 9:14. A
Noahide who kills by accident may also be put to death by the blood
avenger: see *Sifra, Deut.* 19, no. 180; Maimonides, *Hil. Melakhim*
10:1, cf. *Guide for the Perplexed* 3:40 in which the blood avenger is
cited in addition to the king as an agency for punishing murderers
who are not executed by the court.

95. The general jurisdiction of the Israelite monarch is derived from
Deut. 17; 1 *Sam.* 8: see Blidstein, *op. cit.,* ch. 7 for an extensive
analysis of this general jurisdiction. Another relevant general
concept is the principle. 'The law of the land is law' *(dina
demalkhuta dina)* which is normally associated with non-Jewish
kings: see S. Shilo, *Dina Demalkhuta Dina* (Jerusalem, 5735) for a
comprehensive study of this principle.

96. *Or Sameah, Hil. Melakhim* 3:10, cf. Meiri, *Sanh.* 57b, and see
Blidstein, *op. cit.* p.131.

97. This would certainly seem to be the case in relation to theft and
robbery in the view of R. Joseph Albo, see n.50. Also see *B.M.* 61b
for a Talmudic source implying that theft is an offence which could
be derived from reason alone, and see Rashi, *ad loc.*

98. See Blidstein, *op cit.,* p.124, notes 18, 19, who cites these sources,
but doubts whether this category extends beyond the offence of
bloodshed. An opposing view is adopted by R. David Bleich,
Contemporary Halakhic Problems 2 (New York, 1983) p. 351 n.11. In
the final analysis the issue turns on the legal significance of passages
which are prima facie of a legendary rather than legal nature.

99. *Hemdat Yisrael* 1, *Kuntres Ner Mitzvah* no. 288, p. 75; Bleich, *op.
cit.,* p.352, n.11. An allusion to the king's jurisdiction to punish those
guilty of sexual licentiousness is found in *Y. Sanh.* 6:3; see also
Radbaz, *Hil. Melakhim* 3:10.

100. Maimonides, *Hil. Sanhedrin* 18-6; *Or Sameah, Hil. Mealkhim* 3:10;
R. Meir Malbim, *Dvar Shmuel,* 2 *Sam.* 12:5. Also see n.66.

101. See R. Joseph Cohen, *'Dina Demalkhuta* and the improvement of
society' (Heb.), *Hatorah Vehamedinah* 1 (5709) 21; R. Saul Yisraeli,
'The legal jurisdiction of the monarchy in contemporary times'
(Heb.), *Hatorah Vehamedinah* 2 (5710), 80 n.2, 88; R. Judah
Gershuni, 'The Law of the Sanhedrin and the monarchy and the
difference between them', *Hatorah Vehamedinah* 2 (5710), 72; see
also Blidstein, *op. cit.,* p.127.

102. See n. 90. Blidstein, *op. cit.,* n.25 draws attention to a *responsum* of
R. Joseph ibn Migash no. 191, according to which the rubric of
'emergency measures' is restricted to cases in which a person had
committed the offence in question on a number of occasions, or the
offence had spread throughout society. Also see R. Judah Gershuni,
Mishpat Hamelukhah (Jerusalem, 5740), 96, who argues that
whereas the court is restricted to 'emergency measures', the king
can introduce legislation in order to preserve society.

103. *Hil. Melakhim* 3:10; Gershuni, *id.,* cf. R. Zvi Hayyes, *Torat Neviim,*
ch. 7 in *Kol Kitvei Maharaz Hayyes* 1 (Jerusalem, 5718), 49; R. Issac
Herzog, 'The king's right to pardon convicted offenders in Jewish
law' (Heb.), *Hatorah Vehamedinah* 1 (5709), 18.

104. In this respect, it is interesting to compare the king's extra-judicial role in the *halakhah* with the position of Islamic law. The latter system also recognises that the king was empowered to give effect to the general purposes of God for Islamic society, even if this entailed overriding the strict provisions of Islamic law and procedure. In pursuing these purposes, the sovereign was afforded an overriding personal discretion to determine, according to time and circumstances, how the purposes of God for the Islamic community might best be effected. From a comparative perspective, the following excerpt from N. Coulson, *A History of Islamic Law* (Edinburgh, 1964), pp.132-3 is particularly noteworthy:

> It is the criminal law, perhaps, which affords the outstanding instance of the wide discretionary powers granted to the sovereign under the doctrine of *siyasa shaariya*. As far as concerns procedure, he may order the use of such methods as he sees fit to discover where guilt lies, for as one author states, 'were we simply to subject each suspect to the oath and then free him, in spite of our knowledge of his notoriety in crime, saying, We cannot convict him without two upright witnesses, that would be contrary to *siyasa shaariya* . . . ' he may punish at his discretion persons who have committed homicides or assaults when they have been pardoned by the victim or his representatives.

On the prominent role of the king, in maintaining Islam, see: E. Rosenthal, 'Some aspects of Islamic political thought', *Islamic Culture* 22 (1948), 1. The development of the king's role as the principle agency for the maintenance of Islam in Muslim law is traced by J. Schacht, 'The law', in *Unity and Variety in Muslim Civilisation,* ed. G. von Grunebaum, (Chicago, 1985), p.71.

105. *Hemdat Yisrael* 1, *Kuntres Ner Mitzvah* no. 288 p.75.

106. See n.43.

107. On the effect of the rational nature of the Noahide laws on the evidentiary and procedural requirements of the criminal law, see n.68.

108. See *Resp. Mishpat Kohen* no. 144; R. Saul Yisraeli, 'The authority of the president and the elected governmental institutions in the State of Israel', (Heb.), *Hatorah vehamedinah* 1 (5709), 76; and see Elon, *op. cit.,* pp.1, 42; cf. R. Benjamin Teumin Rabinowitz, 'Capital offences under the law of the Sanhedrin and of the king respectively' (Heb.), *Hatorah Vehamedinah* 4 (5712), 79; and R. Yisraeli's response on p.82.

109. See A. Wiesbard, 'On the bioethics of Jewish law: the case of Karen Quinlan', *Israel Law Review* 14 (1979), 359.

110. See the leading case of *R. v. Dudley and Stephens* (1884) 14 QBD 273; A. Simpson, *Cannibalism and the Common Law* (Penguin, 1986), p.248; and below, ch. 3, second section.

111. See n.72.

112. See ch. 3, p.59 below for further discussion of this point.

113. See n.74.

3

SACRIFICING THE LIFE OF A *TEREFAH* FOR THE SAKE OF PRESERVING VIABLE LIFE

According to some authorities, it is permitted to sacrifice the life of a *terefah* for the sake of preserving viable life.[1] In the first section of the chapter, the legal basis for this view will be explored, and the conditions under which it becomes operative will be defined. The following section is concerned with diminished viability as a general principle for choosing between lives in the *halakhah*. The third section deals with the defence of necessity to a murder charge in English common law, and compares it with the halakhic position regarding the killing of a *terefah*. In the final section some of the moral ramifications of recognising diminished viability as an operative legal factor will be discussed in the light of the previous comparative section.

The Legal Basis for Permitting the Sacrifice of a Terefah for the Sake of Saving a Viable Life

The basic principle in Jewish law is that the life of one individual cannot be sacrificed for the sake of another. The source for this principle is the Talmudic dictum 'How do you know that your blood is redder? Perhaps the blood of the other person is redder?'[2] On the basis of this principle, the rule is derived that martyrdom should be chosen in a case in which the only other option is to commit murder.[3] If many lives are at stake, however, the position is not so simple, and this principle may be modified to a certain extent. The classic case of this type of situation in Jewish legal literature is that of a group of travellers threatened by brigands, and given the choice between death and delivering up one of their number to the slaughter. According to the *Tosefta*,[4] the person concerned may be handed over, provided that a specific request was made for that person. This provision is immediately qualified. According to one view, the specified individual may only be delivered up if the whole group is faced with certain death.[5] Under another view, he may only be sacrificed if he is guilty of a crime.[6] Maimonides rules in accordance with the second view and the majority of commentators follow this ruling.[7] Thus, the specified individual may not be handed over unless he is guilty of a criminal, or possibly moral, offence.[8]

Would the position be any different if the group contained a *terefah?* In his commentary on the *Talmud,* R. Menahem Meiri refers to this *Tosefta* and makes the following observations with regard to this contingency:

> It goes without saying that in the case of a group of travellers, if one of them was a *terefah* he may be surrendered in order to save the lives of the rest, since the killer of a *terefah* is exempt from the death penalty.[9]

According to R. Meiri, then, the fact that killing a *terefah* does not entail capital punishment indicates that his life does not possess the same value as that of a viable person in a case in which many lives might be saved as a result of his death. In this respect, the exemption of the killer of a *terefah* from the death penalty is not only a technical requirement of the rules governing the administration of capital punishment; it also serves as a basis for determining the inferior status of a *terefah* as a living person in a situation in which viable life is at stake.

The conceptual basis for R. Meiri's position is articulated by a later authority, R. Joseph Babad, who argues that a *terefah* may be sacrificed for the sake of saving viable lives on the grounds that his blood is indeed 'less red' than that of a healthy individual.[10] As already observed, the prohibition on sacrificing one life for the sake of another is based upon the rational principle of one life being no 'less red' than another. In the case of a *terefah,* however, it is clear that by virtue of the fatal disease from which he is suffering, his life is indeed 'less red' than that of a viable individual. In purely rational terms, therefore, there is no valid reason for preserving the life of a *terefah* when the lives of viable individuals are at stake.

A significant challenge to this view is mounted by R. Ezekiel Landau, one of the outstanding halakhic authorities of the eighteenth century. According to R. Landau, the fact that there is no capital punishment for taking the life of a *terefah* does not mean that he can be killed for the sake of saving a viable person: 'The very idea that a *terefah* might be killed for the sake of preserving a viable life is unheard of'.[11] The correct solution in a conflict situation of this type is, in R. Landau's view, to 'sit and do nothing',[12] since the obligation to save life is not strong enough to override the 'prohibition on the direct killing of a *terefah*' which is derived from the offence of bloodshed, as explained in the previous chapter.[13]

This solution, however, is criticised by a later authority, R. Isaac Schmelkes, according to whom it is arguable that the passivity rule only applies to positive commandments affecting Jews. It does not apply to paramount obligations such as the saving of human life, which is binding upon both Jews and Noahides. The fact that the killer of a *terefah* is exempt from the death penalty also means that the negative prohibition in this case is not a strong one. Where there is a choice between a *terefah* and a viable person, therefore, the latter ought to be preferred.[14]

R. Schmelkes's view is in turn criticised by R. Ovadia Yosef, who maintains that the categorisation of the obligation to save life as a paramount one, and hence outside the ambit of the passivity rule, is a debatable point. R. Yosef also observes that the argument from the absence of capital punishment with respect to the killing of a *terefah* is not a justification for reducing him to an inferior status in a situation of conflict with a viable individual.[15]

There would, however, appear to be a basic distinction between the cases considered by R. Meiri and R. Landau, respectively, which may very well make it unnecessary to reach any definite conclusion as to which of the two views is definitive.[16] In the case of the travellers threatened by a band of brigands dealt with by R. Meiri, the issue is clearly one of indirect homicide, i.e. handing over one of the travellers to a killer. R. Landau's comments were made in relation to the question of destroying a foetus in order to save its mother's life. The actual point with which R. Landau is concerned is Maimonides's reference to the pursuer principle in his codification of the Mishnaic ruling that before a foetus may be destroyed for the sake of preserving maternal life.[17] Not only is the application of this principle in the context of foeticide specifically rejected by the *Talmud* but even on purely logical grounds the same result could have been achieved in a more direct fashion by simply contrasting the fact that capital punishment is imposed for the murder of the mother, whereas destruction of the foetus carries no penalty whatsoever in the criminal law. In order to defend Maimonides's reliance upon the pursuer principle in the context of abortion, R. Landau must demonstrate that the absence of a specific criminal sanction on foeticide cannot by itself serve as a justification for performing an abortion for the sake of the mother, and he does so on the basis of the total unacceptability of this argument in the context of the *terefah*. He is dealing, therefore, with a direct act of killing, namely foeticide. It is not at all obvious that his objection to killing a *terefah* for the sake of viable life would also apply to a case such as that of the travellers, in which the issue is indirect homicide. In such a case, even R. Landau might admit that the *terefah* could be handed over for the sake of the rest of the group.[18]

In the light of this distinction, it is arguable that the *halakhah* would permit the indirect killing of a *terefah* in order to save viable life. The question of determining indirectness is governed by the ordinary principles of causation in Jewish law.[19] In the context of the treatment of the critically ill, it has been argued that disconnecting an artificial respirator from a comatose vegetative patient by means of a time switch constitutes an indirect method of terminating treatment.[20] On this basis, it would appear that the availability of sophisticated medical technology for the treatment of different types of critical illness may at the same time provide a suitable framework for justifying the termination of the lives of such patients in circumstances mandated by the relevant halakhic categories.[21]

The final question which must be considered in this section is the number[22] of lives which must be at risk in order to justify the indirect killing of a *terefah*. In the light of R. Babad's argument that the life of a *terefah* is 'less red' than that of a viable person, there would appear to be no logical basis for distinguishing between the number of viable lives at stake. In fact, R. Babad himself maintains that when faced with the choice between martyrdom and the murder of a *terefah*, the latter course of action is the one to be preferred.[23] It may, therefore, be concluded that according to the views of R. Meiri and R. Babad, there would be no objection to sacrificing a *terefah* for the sake of saving viable life, provided that the method of causing death was an indirect one. Indeed, this is the conclusion reached by R. Judah Gershuni in an essay on the issue of heart transplants in the *halakhah*.[24] According to R. Gershuni, removing a heart from a *terefah* donor would be permitted by R. Meiri 'and those following his views', on the basis of the above-mentioned argument, notwithstanding that it is the life of only one viable individual which is at stake. It is also noteworthy that the fact that the donee in this case is only viable by virtue of the heart which is available for transplanting does not make him a non-viable individual. Clearly, the non-viability of human *tarfut* is to be determined on the basis of both actual and potential factors. This line of argument has been developed in recent writings on the halakhic feasibility of heart transplants, and may very well have influenced the recent decision by the Israeli Chief Rabbinate to permit heart transplants under Jewish law.[25]

The diminished viability of the *terefah* is, therefore, a significant factor in situations in which a choice must be made between his life and that of another person. Where no such choice is required, the diminished viability of the *terefah* is immaterial: his killer is classified as a shedder of blood and is liable to divine and extra-legal penalties. In the following section, the role played by diminished viability in deciding between the lives of foetuses and newly born babies and viable individuals or groups will be examined and compared with the position in relation to the *terefah*.

Diminished Viability as a General Principle in Situations Involving a Choice Between Lives

In the previous chapter, it was observed that foeticide is not a capital crime in Jewish law. It was also demonstrated that since foeticide does carry the death penalty under the Noahide code, it is prohibited to Israelites and may very well carry a divine sanction.[26] In this respect, there is a striking similarity between the source and nature of the prohibition on unjustified foeticide, and killing a *terefah;* i.e. both are derived from the Noahide offence of bloodshed and both carry divine and/or extra-legal penalties.

As far as the question of sacrificing a foetus for the sake of its mother's life is concerned, the halakhic position is quite definitive. According to the *Mishnah,* if a woman's life is threatened in childbirth and the only way to save her is to kill the foetus, then 'her life takes precedence.'[27] If the baby has been born, as defined by the emergence of the head in the case of a normal birth[28] and the protrusion of the majority of the body in a Caesarian delivery,[29] Then 'the life of one person does not override that of another'.[30] From the Mishnaic ruling, it is clear that only after birth does a foetus become a person, and his murderer becomes liable to capital punishment. The reason for preferring the life of the mother to that of the foetus is, therefore, that the latter is not yet a person.[31] According to many authorities, the proof of this proposition lies in the fact that under biblical law, a person who causes a woman to miscarry must pay her husband for the loss of his offspring, but he is not liable to any further sanction.[32] In this respect, the position regarding therapeutic abortion is similar to the *halakhah* in relation to sacrificing a *terefah* for the sake of saving viable life, i.e. the nexus between lack of sanction and permission to sacrifice life in situations of conflict with viable beings.[33]

There are, nevertheless, some obvious differences between the two cases. As already observed, a *terefah* may only be killed in an indirect fashion, whereas a foetus which is threatening the life of its mother may be destroyed in a direct manner.[34] On the other hand, while a *terefah* may be sacrificed for the sake of any viable life, permission to abort a foetus would appear to be restricted to the one case of saving the mother's life. According to R. Babad, however, the same principle underlying the permission to sacrifice a *terefah* for the sake of viable life would also apply to a foetus, i.e. the blood of a foetus is indeed 'less red' than that of a viable individual.[35] Hence, in any conflict situation involving a foetus, viable life takes precedence. Indeed, such conclusion was reached by R. Isser Unterman in a case which arose in the course of the German occupation of Lithuania during the First World War, in which a German physician ordered a Jewish doctor to perform an abortion or be killed. According to R. Unterman, martyrdom is not required in such a case, since there is no specific biblical prohibition on foeticide.[36] It would appear, therefore, that the confinement of the issue of justified foeticide to the context of conflict between foetal life and maternal life is merely a reflection of reality: in the ordinary course of events it is this conflict, rather than any other, that is likely to arise for consideration.

It is arguable that the first difference observed above (the fact that a *terefah,* unlike a foetus, may be killed only indirectly) is attributable to the side-effects of the deed rather than the deed itself. Clearly, the effect upon society of the direct killing of a *terefah* who is capable of 'eating, drinking and walking about on the streets' is much more traumatic than that of directly destroying a foetus which is threatening the mother's life. Indeed, the strong rhetorical language used by R. Ezekiel Landau in his objection to the idea that a *terefah* could be sacrificed for the sake of a viable person[37] would appear to support this contention. It will also be recalled that this objection constitutes the main basis for his requirement of indirectness in the case of a *terefah*. In this light, the difference in relation to the issue of indirectness would seem to be rather insignificant in comparison with the striking similarities between the *terefah* and the foetus as outlined above.

A further similarity between the *terefah* and the foetus emerges in the context of the Sabbath laws. The idea that a *terefah* could be killed in a direct fashion in order to save viable life was dismissed by R. Ezekield Landau on various grounds, one of which was that the Sabbath may be desecrated in order to preserve the life of a person who has only a short time to live.[38] The implication of this argument is that the Sabbath may be profaned in order to save the life of a *terefah*. This, however, is open to question, since the *Talmud* implies that the Sabbath may not be profaned in order to save an infant of doubtful viability.[39] Although it is arguable that this Talmudic source is referring to 'desecration' of the Sabbath by performing a circumcision rather than to the saving of life,[40] there is nevertheless a solid body of opinion to the effect that it does, in fact, refer to general life-saving treatment.[41] In the final analysis, therefore, the saving of a *terefah's* life at the cost of desecrating the Sabbath is a moot point.

Violation of the Sabbath for the sake of saving foetal life is also a moot point. The Talmudic ruling to the effect that the Sabbath may be profaned in order to bring a knife to cut open the womb of a dead woman and take out her child[42] would appear to be confined to cases in which the mother is already dead and the foetus is considered as a separate and independent entity.[43] The issue of saving foetal life *per se* is, therefore, a matter of debate. According to one view, the Sabbath may not be violated since the foetus is not a person.[44] Another view holds that the Sabbath may be desecrated for the sake of the foetus on the grounds that in the future the foetus will grow into a person who will observe many Sabbaths.[45] It is, however, widely held that, in practice, it is impossible to differentiate between a threat to the life of the foetus and to that of the mother.[46] Since there is no doubt that the Sabbath can be profaned on the mother's behalf, the question of profaning it on behalf of the foetus becomes irrelevant. This, it is suggested, is the reason for the omission of any reference to the question of desecrating the

Sabbath for the sake of foetal life in any of the standard codes of Jewish law.[47] Thus, in the final analysis, even the view which does permit the Sabbath to be desecrated for the sake of saving the life of a foetus does so on the basis of its future potential, and not on the basis of its present status. The lack of physical development characteristic of both the *terefah* and the foetus is, therefore, an operative issue in the area of the Sabbath laws.[48] Since neither the *terefah* nor the foetus are considered as full persons in Jewish law, the Sabbath may not necessarily be broken for the sake of preserving their lives.

Another area in which doubts are raised as to the applicability of the principle that one life may not be sacrificed for the sake of another is the killing of a non-viable infant. Although a foetus becomes a person at birth,[49] human viability is determined by other criteria. According to the *Talmud,* a human being is not presumed to be viable unless he fulfils one of two conditions: either thirty days have elapsed since birth, or a full nine months have elapsed between conception and birth.[50] As in the case of the *terefah,* the death penalty ought not to be imposed for the murder of a non-viable child, since in capital cases, the accused always receives the benefit of the doubt.[51] The question arises, however, of the determination of viability in the case of a child under the age of thirty days. According to one view, it is virtually impossible to ascertain whether exactly nine months have passed since conception or not. As a result, the killer receives the benefit of the doubt, and may not be executed.[52] Although there is a Mishnaic ruling to the effect that the killer of a one-day old child is liable to the death penalty,[53] this ruling is of theoretical significance only.[54] The opposite view maintains that it is ordinarily assumed that every birth occurs exactly nine months after conception, and that as a result, the murderer of a newly born infant will be subject to capital punishment unless he can show that the ordinary presumption is incorrect in his case.[55] Viability is, therefore, a factor in determining whether or not the murderer of a newly born child is to be executed.

It is on this basis that R. David Hoffman argues that it is permitted to sacrifice a newly born child in order to preserve the life of its mother.[56] His reason is the doubtful viability of the child, which does indeed make his blood 'less red' than that of its mother. Other authorities also permit the sacrifice of the child in these circumstances, but base their ruling upon the principle of specification mentioned above.[57] According to these authorities, the very fact that a newly born child poses a threat to its mother's life is sufficient grounds for treating it as a specified individual whose life may be sacrificed for the sake of saving viable life.[58]

It would appear, however, that R. Hoffman's approach is a better one. First, it has been argued that the specification principle is inapplicable in cases of this nature since, *inter alia,* divine providence may yet bring about the salvation of both mother and offspring by removing the cause of the threat to the life of the former.[59] Secondly, adoption of R. Hoffman's reasoning in this context would also resolve other difficulties, such as the fact that in this case there is only one life at stake, i.e. that of the mother, whereas in the case of the group of travellers, many lives are in jeopardy.[60] On the view that the crucial issue is that of viability, however, this would not constitute a difficulty, since it has already been established in relation to the *terefah* that the principle of the blood of a non-viable individual being 'less red' than that of a viable person does indeed apply on a one-to-one basis.[61]

In R. Hoffman's view, therefore, there is a clear link between non-viability and permission to sacrifice a newly born infant for the sake of saving viable life. In this respect, it is noteworthy that in theory the Sabbath ought not to be profaned for the sake of a non-viable child.[62] This ruling is obviously another manifestation of the link between viability and legal status in situations of conflict with other values.

The conclusion flowing from this discussion is that diminished viability does indeed constitute a basis for preferring one life over another, and for preserving the Sabbath at the expense of human life. In principle, therefore, Jewish law does recognise a biological criterion for evaluating human life in situations where one life can only be saved at the expense of another.

In practice, it is clear that this criterion becomes operative only in very limited circumstances. There is no question of terminating a viability-deficient life in any situation other than that of saving a viable one. Present or future suffering is not by itself sufficient grounds for terminating a life of deficient viability.

It is also necessary to observe that the means used for the actual termination of life in these circumstances is normally required to be of an indirect, rather than a direct, nature. This point has already been made in relation to the *terefah,* and since the sacrifice of a newly born infant is based on the same reasoning (i.e. his blood is indeed 'less red' than that of a viable individual) it may be concluded that the indirectness requirement also applies to the newly born. In the case of the foetus, various authorities have ruled that only in the most urgent case should direct means of abortion be used. In the first instance, indirect means are preferable.[63] In any case, at the prima-facie level,[64] justifiable foeticide is confined to saving the life of the mother.

It must also be emphasised that the mandate to preserve the Sabbath at the expense of a human life of diminished viability is of theoretical interest only. In practice, all cases involving such deficient forms of life would be treated as doubtful cases, with the result that no effort would be spared to save such life even at the expense of the sanctity of the Sabbath.[65]

Nevertheless, there are certain cases in which the link between deficient viability and the saving of one life at the expense of another did, in fact, become an operative one in Jewish law. A number of such cases can be found in halakhic *responsa* relating to episodes which took place during the Holocaust. In one such case, a group of Jews were hiding from the Nazis when the cries of a baby threatened to reveal their presence to the German soldiers who were searching the area in which they were concealed. The baby was smothered to death in order to prevent its cries from attracting the attention of the Nazis. This action was justified by R. Simon Efrati, with some reservations concerning the correctness of such action on a spiritual level.[66] The special circumstances of this case also emerge from the fact that the killing was sanctioned even though it was effected in a direct manner.

Another case of this genre is cited in an article devoted to cases arising in the Holocaust.[67] The case considered is that of throwing the victims of the Nazi gas chambers into crematoria, notwithstanding that they still exhibit some signs of life. It is suggested that the non-viable condition of the victims, together with the threat of certain death hanging over those ordered to dispose of the corpses should they not do so, would justify a halakhic decision in favour of permitting a Jewish worker to throw such corpses into the crematoria.[68]

It is, therefore, evident that diminished viability is a general principle in Jewish law in the context of tragic choices such as those outlined above. In the following section, this principle will be compared with the position regarding the defence of necessity to a murder charge in the common law of England. The fourth and final section of the chapter is concerned with the moral image of the *halakhah* in this area.

The Defence of Necessity and the Crime of Murder in English Common Law

At first sight, it might appear that in permitting the sacrifice of a *terefah* for the sake of saving viable life, the *halakhah* adopts a lower moral standard than other legal systems, and in particular, the common law of England in which no such exception to the principle of the inviolability of human life is recognised. The object of the present section is to demonstrate that although English common law does not formally recognise this type of necessity as a defence to a murder charge, it does, nevertheless, treat such cases more leniently than ordinary cases of homicide.

The leading case in this area is undoubtedly that of *R*. v. *Dudley and Stephens* (1884) 14 QBD 273.[69] In this case, three men and a body of the crew of a yacht were shipwrecked. After eighteen days in an open boat, having been without food and water for several days, the two accused suggested killing the boy and eating him. Two days later, Stephens killed the boy, who at this stage was extremely weak. The three men then fed on the boy's flesh, and four days later they were rescued. The accused were indicted for murder (the third mariner turned Queen's evidence).[70] The jury, by special verdict, found that the men would probably have died within the four days had they not fed on the boy's body, that the boy would probably have died before them and that, at the time of the killing, there was no appreciable chance of saving life, except by killing one for the others to eat. The accused were convicted of murder, but the death sentence was commuted to six months imprisonment.

The defence raised by the accused to the murder charge was that of necessity. This defence was rejected by the court on the following grounds:

> Who is to be the judge of this sort of necessity? By what measure is the comparative value of lives to be measured? Is it to be strength or intellect or what? It is plain that the principle [of necessity] leaves to him who is to profit by it

to determine the necessity which will justify him in deliberately taking another's life to save his own.[71]

The common law does not, therefore, recognise the principle of necessity in the context of the crime of murder.

The basic position of the common law would thus appear to correspond to that of the *halakhah* which, in principle, refuses to determine whether or not the blood of one man is 'redder' than that of another. The difference between the two systems emerges only with respect to controversial cases. Whereas the *halakhah* specifies exceptions to its basic position, e.g. the principles drawn from the case of the travellers cited in the *Tosefta* and the exemption of the killer of a *terefah* from the death penalty, the common law does not. Possible exceptions are raised by learned authors,[72] but the definitive position is undoubtedly the one summed up in the following extract:

> When, however, all is said and done, probably the most persistent English attitude to the problem raised by the necessity plea—intellectually unsatisfying though it may be—is that hard cases are best dealt with by the prerogative of mercy.[73]

Indeed, in *R.* v. *Dudley and Stephens* itself, the death sentence for murder was commuted to six months imprisonment.

A striking feature of this strategy is that the common law is capable of maintaining an uncompromisingly negative attitude towards the idea of choosing between lives while at the same time leaving room for morally extenuating circumstances to be taken into account at the post-trial or executive level. It is possible that the notion of the sanctity of life in the Christian tradition[74] and the primacy of the value of life in Natural law thinking[75] both provide the historical basis for this uncompromising attitude towards choosing between lives that is characteristic of the common law. In any case, it is undoubtedly this attitude which underlies the popularity of the wedge principle argument against any form of euthanasia amongst scholars writing in the common law tradition.[76] According to this argument, no dilution of the primacy of the value of human life in the legal system can be tolerated, since any such dilution inevitably leads to the totally unjustifiable destruction of human lives. [77] It is against this background that declarations such as that of B. Cardozo to the effect that the courts will not recognise a 'principle of human jettison' in cases such as *R.* v. *Dudley and Stephens* were made.[78]

Clearly, this is not a feature shared by the *halakhah*. This difference between Jewish law, which is prepared to recognise exceptions to the supremacy of human life within the context of the substantive criminal law, and other systems which are not, was noticed by R. Solomon Duran and was utilised by him in a polemical work in defence of the *Talmud*.[79] In comparing the *halakhah's* exemption of the killer of a *terefah* from the death penalty, with the secular law in which there is no such provision, R. Duran observes that the use of the royal pardon in offences of this kind in secular law parallels the exemption of the *terefah* in the *halakhah*. The two systems, therefore, accept the basic principle that the killer of a non-viable individual is not subjected to the full penal rigours of the criminal law, but adopt different strategies in applying the principle within the system. Jewish law recognises specific exceptions to capital punishment and the offence of murder, whereas the gentile law referred to by R. Duran and English common law rely upon royal pardons in order to achieve the same effect. The different strategies undoubtedly arise from underlying distinctions between the two systems and it is to this issue that the final section of this chapter is devoted.

Underlying Moral Differences between Jewish and Common Law

It has already been established that the basic exemption of the killer of a *terefah* from capital punishment is complemented by the existence of a prohibition on bloodshed, and the imposition of divine and extra-legal sanctions. The entrenchment of the concept of the fundamental value of human life in a society based upon Jewish law is, therefore, carried out by means of powerful institutions within the *halakhah*,[80] although capital punishment is not one of them. This is not the case with regard to the common law, at least not in the modern period. In the light of the absence of such institutions in the common law, it is clear that it would, in moral terms, risk much greater moral losses by ameliorating the absolute prohibition on choosing between lives in this type of situation than does the *halakhah*. This difference between the two systems is highly significant in any attempt to gain a better understanding of the moral image of the *halakhah* in this area of the law, and will indeed be examined further in the next chapter.

Another significant difference between the two systems which might account for their different strategies with respect to choosing between lives is rather more historical than substantive.

The *halakhah,* as already observed, is characterised by the existence of a 'well-established framework of primary and secondary principles, and a long history of highly refined casuistical thinking'.[81] The halakhist is able to draw upon a wide range of legal distinctions applicable to this issue, all of which are well within the tradition in which he is working. Modern common law, on the other hand, does not possess such a framework, possibly because issues of this nature were, in the past, a matter for religious doctrine, and the question of choosing between lives is too critical for courts to deal with merely on the basis of legislation. Common law, therefore, also lacks a tradition of resolving this type of problem in practical terms. The apparent adherence of the common law to the principle of the supreme value of every human life in an area such as euthanasia is, therefore, also understandable as a manifestation of the absence of any suitable conceptual tool for dealing with this issue. The absence of this type of framework may also explain the preference of the common law for the resolution of hard cases, such as those involving choosing between lives, in procedural rather than substantive terms, i.e. the prerogative of mercy and the general practice of not prosecuting medical personnel involved in terminating the lives of the critically ill. Whatever the merits or demerits of this approach,[82] it constitutes a second important difference between the common law and the *halakhah* with regard to issues of the type under discussion in the present chapter.

In the light of these remarks, it is clear that the *halakhah,* unlike other systems, is not concerned with the dangers of the wedge principle in this area of the law. As already observed, this principle consists of the argument that if the termination of any human life is permitted, then mass slaughter of human beings is the inevitable result. The adherents of the wedge principle argue that if it is permitted to disconnect a device such as an artificial respirator from a patient with absolutely no hope of recovery, the result must inevitably be the extermination of all unwanted members of society by those who have the power and the authority to order their deaths. Hence, no attempt should be made to terminate any form of treatment, including artificial respiration, until the patient's death has been clearly established and vertified. It should be noted that for the purposes of the following discussion, no distinction will be made between different types of life-terminating acts, the assumption being such such distinctions are irrelevant to the moral basis upon which this principle rests.

The wedge principle takes two forms; one logical and the other empirical. The logical form is based on the assumption that killing in any form is an absolute prohibition. Thus, no life-terminating act may be excluded from the prohibition, and if it is transgressed in one case, the way is open for it to be transgressed in others. In this view, there is no room for any distinction in terms of the intention and the consequences in the circumstances of any particular case.[83] Another view of this form of the principle, however, permits such a distinction to be made, and in a case in which there are good reasons for doing so, e.g. if it is the kindest possible course of action for the person concerned, then euthanasia should be allowed. There is thus no necessary logical connection between switching off a respirator and committing mass murder, provided that a clear separation is made, theoretically at least, between killing for a legitimate motive and killing for an illegitimate one.[84] Clearly, the logical form of the wedge principle is at variance with the provisions of Jewish law regarding both *gesisah* and *tarfut,* which theoretically permit the termination of human life in various situations and within certain limits. It is noteworthy that according to one prominent Jewish thinker, these provisions are indeed not in accordance with what he believes to be the moral position of Judaism, i.e. that any form of killing is an absolute prohibition. In order to resolve this contradiction between *halakhah* and morality, he suggests that the provisions concerning *gesisah* and *tarfut* be treated as *halakhah* which is kept concealed from the public because of its potentially negative effect upon public standards of morality and religion, and in these particular cases, upon the fundamental moral value of human life.[85] However, it is very doubtful whether the halakhic rubric in question (that of concealed rules) really covers a situation of this nature, and whether the moral position of Judaism can be successfully dislocated from the halakhic one.[86] In any case, this view is clearly rejected by the majority of halakhists who publish quite openly and widely in this field. Consequently, it is only the empirical view of the wedge principle that now remains to be considered.

The empirical form of the principle is usually linked to the thesis that the Nazi extermination camps had their origins in the euthanasia programme initiated early in the days of the Third

Reich.[87] Accordingly, it is maintained that any form of terminating life will lead to more active killing for the worst possible sorts of reasons. Now, although this thesis is debatable (in the sense that the protection and purification of the Aryan stock rather than humanitarian considerations may very well have been the real motive for this programme from the beginning,[88] it is clear that the Nazi experience teaches a very important lesson about the possible misuse of any type of euthanasia legislation. The real question, however, is whether this lesson is a political rather than a purely legal one. Surely, the moral of the story is that any government that condones death camps is an intolerable government, irrespective of the process by which such camps might have been helped into existence![89]

In any case, even if it were accepted that the empirical wedge principle was borne out by human experience, the point must be made that in Jewish law any attempt to sanction the termination of a human life is controlled by a well-developed body of guiding principles and the threat of divine and external penalties. As a result, the basic premise of the wedge principle, i.e. that the sanctioning of the termination of non-viable life opens up the field to mass killing, is less than convincing. The wedge principle would, in fact, appear to be more appropriate in relation to a society in which the one social institution protecting human life is the positive law. In such a society, the fear that even a slight erosion of this law will eventually lead to the sanctioning of wide-scale murder may be well-founded.[90] In a society operating with the type of system exemplified by the *halakhah,* however, such a fear seems to have little basis. The complex interrelationship of substantive rules and institutional frameworks which characterises this area of the law ensures that the erosion of the primacy of human life by halakhic recognition of diminished viability in situations of conflict between lives does not place society directly on the path to moral chaos.

To sum up, it would appear that where the indirect termination of the life of a critically ill patient would result in the saving of a viable life, as in the case of organ transplants or the allocation of scarce medical resources, Jewish law would, in principle, legitimate such an act, provided that an institutional framework existed for assessing the effect of such a deed upon the moral fabric of society and for administering discretionary punishments. In all cases involving the killing, either directly or indirectly, of a *terefah*, the killer would be exempt from the death penalty and his fate would be decided by extra-judicial bodies. These bodies would have at their disposal a whole range of sanctions, including death. Presumably, where proof was brought to the effect that the death of the *terefah* had been brought about in an indirect fashion for the sake of saving viable life, those involved in the relevant acts would not be subject to any sanction.

Two major issues now arise. The first is the extent to which the *terefah* category figures in contemporary halakhic literature on the question of the treatment of the critically ill. The second is the question of whether or not human *tarfut* is relevant to the question of mercy-killing, and the significance of pain and suffering for the *halakhah* governing the treatment of the dying. Both questions will be examined in the following chapters.

Notes

1. The question of whether or not sacrificing extends to direct killing is discussed below. The majority opinion is that only indirect killing is permitted. In the context of a terminally ill patient, however, the scope for terminating life in an indirect fashion is sufficiently wide to make this view an important one even if it only extends to an indirect act.

2. *Sanh.* 74a.

3. Maimonides, *Hil, Yesodei Hatorah* 5:7; *Shulhan Arukh, Yoreh Deah* 157:1.

4. *T. Ter.* 7:20; S. Leiberman, *Tosefta Kifshutah, Ter.* 7, 148 cf. *Y. Ter.* 8:4; *Gen. Rabbah* 94:9 and *Lev. Rabbah* 19:6. For a general discussion of these sources see D. Daube, *Collaboration with Tyranny in Rabbinic Law* (London, 1965). The main legal distinctions arising out of these sources are discussed by S. Shilo, 'Sacrificing one life for the sake of saving many lives' (Heb.), *Hevra Vehistoriah* (Jerusalem, 5740), 57.

5. cf. *Y. Ter.* 8:4 and Daube, *id.* and Shilo, *id.*

6. *Hil. Yesodei Hatorah* 5:5. The basis for this ruling is discussed in *Kesef Mishneh, Hil. Yesodei Hatorah* 5:5; *Resp. Habah Hayeshanot* no. 43; *Resp. Seridei Esh* 2 no. 78.

7. *Bah, Tur, Yoreh Deah* 153; *Taz, Shulhan Arukh, Yoreh Deah* 157:7; cf. *Hagahot Hagra, Shulhan Arukh, Yoreh Deah* 157:7; *Resp. Noda Beyehuda* 2, *Yoreh Deah* no. 74.

8. The question arises whether or not the crime of which the individual to be handed over is accused must also be a recognised offence in Jewish law: see *Resp. Habah Hayeshanot* no. 43; *Taz. id.*

9. Meiri, *Sanh.* 74a s.v. *yera'eh li.* Also see *Tiferet Yisrael, Yom.* 8:7 s.v. *venireh li.* The fact that R. Meiri does not extend this provision to *gesisah* provides further evidence that a *goses* is considered as a normal healthy person.

64   Sacrificing a *Terefah* to Preserve Viable Life

10. *Minhat Hinukh* no. 296 *s.v. vehinei beguf hadin.*

11. *Resp. Noda Beyehuda* 2, *Hoshen Mishpat* no. 59.

12. This rule is generally applied with respect to the nullification of positive biblical commandments which are in conflict with Rabbinic prohibitions: see *Ber.* 20a; *Yeb.* 80a; Rashi, *Ber.* 20a *s.v. shev ve'al ta'aseh.*

13. See p.30 above.

14. *Resp. Beth Yitzhak* 2, *Yoreh Deah* no. 162:3.

15. *Resp. Yabia Omer* 4, *Even Haezer* no. 1.

16. In a recent essay on heart transplants in Jewish law, R. Judah Gershuni assumed that the issue remained unresolved. Hence, on the question of removing a heart from a *terefah* for the purpose of a transplant, R. Meiri's school would incline to the permissive view, whereas R. Landau's school would forbid it: see *Kol. Zafayikh* (Jerusalem, 5740), 376. Also see *Tiferet Yisrael, Yom.* 8:7 s.v. *venireh li* for a similar argument.

17. See *Hil. Rozeah* 2:9; *M. Ohol.* 7:6 and *Sanh.* 72b. For a discussion of these sources and the prohibition on foeticide in Jewish law, see p.29 above.

18. This and other distinctions drawn in order to reconcile the two views are dealt with in the following sources: *Resp. Yabia Omer* 4, *Even Haezer* no. 1; R. Benjamin Rabinowitz-Teumim, 'Extradition to non-Jewish authorities', (Heb.), *Noam* 17 (5734), 357. R. Isaiah Karelitz is somewhat ambivalent in his support of the distinction: see *Hazon Ish, Sanh.* no. 25, and note R. Rabinowitz's strong criticism of this ambivalence. Classical sources in which this distinction is made in general terms include *Levush Mordekhai, Yoreh Deah* 157:1 and *Tiferet Yisrael, Yoma* 3:3. Also see Shilo *op. cit.* p. 60; A. Enker, 'Homicide committed in circumstances of duress and necessity in Jewish law', (Heb.) *Shenaton Hamishpat Haivri* 2 (5737), 171; and E. Ben-Zimra, 'Bloodshed by necessity in Jewish law and Israeli law' (Heb.), *Shenaton Hamishpat Haivri* 3–4 (5736–7), 142.

19. See p.31 and 32 above.

20. *Resp. Ziz Eliezer* 13 no. 89.

21. In effect this suggestion is merely a recommendation to restore the status quo which, in fact, is a classical interpretation of the distinction between precipitating death and removing an impediment with respect to a *goses:* see p.12 above.

22. The argument that the number of lives at stake in a case of this nature ought to be a decisive factor is advanced in the context of moral philosophy by J. Harris, *Violence and Responsibility* (London, 1980), ch. 5. According to Harris:

> in any group of three or more dying people where the sacrifice of one would save the other two and where all would die if the sacrifice was not made, then to fail to sacrifice one for two is to kill two people. So long as the choice of who to sacrifice is made fairly [p.81].

However, Harris's view is subject to criticism: see J. Taurek, 'Should the numbers count', *Philosophy and Public Affairs* 6 (1977), 293 on the grounds that 'suffering is not additive'. Also see J. Glover, *Causing Death and Saving Lives* (Penguin, 1981), ch. 16, according to whom it is the issue of side-effects, e.g. the terror in society resulting from the possibility that someone might suddenly have his vital organs forcibly removed for the sake of saving a number of lives, which constitutes the strongest objection to taking numbers into account. In terms of absolute morality, the argument for not taking numbers into account is not such a strong one. In terms of Jewish law, however, the selection is based upon the criterion of *tarfut,* and in this respect, the side-effects are undoubtedly less traumatic since the individual in question is bound to die in any case.

23. *Minhat Hinukh* no. 296 s.v. *vehinei beguf hadin.*
24. See n. 16 above.
25. See Gershuni, op. cit.; R. Mordekhai Halperin, 'Heart transplants according to the halakhah' (Heb.), *Sefer Assia* 5, ed. M. Halperin (Jerusalem, 5746), 68ff. For the decision of the Israeli Chief Rabbinate permitting heart transplants, see: *Assia* 42–3 (5747), 70. The actual decision is based upon the acceptance of brain death as a legitimate definition of death for the purposes of Jewish law, but it is possible that the decision was influenced by earlier articles on the status of the *terefah* and the notion that his diminished viability means that his life may be sacrificed for the sake of a viable, or potentially viable, individual.
26. See p.30 above.
27. *M. Ohol.* 7:6, cf. *T. Arak.* 1:4.
28. See *T. Yeb.* 9:5; *Yeb.* 72b; *Nidd.* 29a; *Y. Sanh.* 8:9; Maimonides, *Hil. Rozeah* 1:9; *Shulhan Arukh, Hoshen Mishpat* 425:2.
29. See *Resp. Melamed Lehoil3* no. 89; *Resp. Panim Meirot* 3 no. 8 and *Pri Ha'adamah, Hil. Nahalot* 1:13.
30. *M. Ohol.* 7:6.
31. Rashi, *Sanh.* 72b s.v. *yatza; Ramban, Nidd.* 44b s.v. *had ditnan;* Ramban, *Torat Ha'adam, Inyan Hasakanah* s.v. *uvahalakhot;* Meiri, *Sanh.* 72b s.v. *ubarah;* Ran. *Hull., ch. 3 (19a) s.v. ulinyan;* Yad Remah, *Sanh.* 72b s.v. *aval kol zeman.* See R. Michael Stern, *Harefuah Leor Hahalakhah* (Jerusalem, 5740), pt 1, sec. 1, ch. 3.
32. *Ex.* 21:22; *Resp. Radbaz Mikhtav Yad* 8 no. 22; Sema, *Hoshen Mishpat* 425:8. Also see R. Moses Zweig, 'Concerning abortion' (Heb.), *Noam* 7 (5724), 39; Stern, *ibid.,* pt 1, sec. 1, ch. 4.
33. Meiri, *Sanh.* 74a s.v. *yera'eh li,* and see above p.50.
34. Maimonides in *Hil. Rozeah* 1:9 observes that the foetus in such a case may be dismembered 'manually or with a potion'. This distinction is interpreted to indicate that both direct and indirect methods may be used in performing a therapeutic abortion: see R. Aryeh Lifshutz, *Aryeh Debei Ilai, Yoreh Deah* no. 19, however, cf. n.63 in which the view that indirect methods should be chosen before direct is cited.
35. *Minhat Hinukh* no. 296 s.v. *vehinei beguf hadin* and see first section above. According to R. Babad, the mother's life is of no greater intrinsic value than that of any other person; hence, if the *Mishnah (Ohol.* 7:6) authorises therapeutic abortion for her sake, foeticide is permitted to save the life of any individual.
36. See R. Unterman, *Shevet Miyehuda* (Jerusalem, 5715), 29 for a full discussion of this case. Also see Stern, *op. cit.,* pt 1, sec. 1, p.77. Incidents involving a choice between smothering an infant and exposing a whole group of Jewish adults to the risk of detection and death at the hands of the Nazis in the Second World War are referred to in the second part of this section.

37. *Resp. Noda Beyehuda* 2 *Hoshen Mishpat* no. 59 and see p.49.
38. *Resp. Noda Beyehuda* 2 *Hoshen Mishpat* no. 59 referring to *Yom.* 85a in which the *Talmud* states that someone buried under a pile of debris should be rescued on the Sabbath day even if 'he has only a short while to live'. Also see Maimonides, *Hil. Shabbat* 2:8; *Shulhan Arukh, Orah Hayyim* 329:4.
39. See *Shab.* 135b; *Shulhan Arukh, Orah Hayyim* 330:8. The question of the status of a newly born infant in the criminal law is fully investigated in the following section.
40. See *Biur Halakhah, Orah Hayyim* 330 s.v. *o safek ben zayin.*
41. *Arukh Hashulhan, Orah Hayyim* 330:13; *Petah Hadevir* 4, *Orah Hayyim* 229.
42. *Arak.* 7a–b.
43. *Tosafot Nidd.* 44b s.v. *ihu;* Ramban, *Torat Ha'adam Inyan Hasakanah* s.v. *ika man disvarah lei.*
44. Ramban, *id.;* Rosh, *Yoma,* ch. 8, no. 13; *Eshkol* 2, *Hil. Milah* no. 36. According to *Magen Avraham, Orah Hayyim* 330:15, this is the definitive view of Ramban,; also see *Resp. Noda Beyehuda* 2 *Hoshen Mishpat* no. 59.
45. *Ba'al Halakhot Gedolot, Hil. Yom Hakipurim* s.v. *ishah ubarah;* Ramban, *Torat Ha'adam, Inyan Hasakanah* s.v. *midekamar mitaker vladah;* Rosh, *Yom.,* ch. 8 no. 13; *Eshkol* 2, *Hil. Milah* no. 36.
46. Rosh, *Yom.,* ch. 8 no. 13; *Korban Netanel, Yom.,* ch. 8, n.20.
47. Stern, *op. cit.,* pt 1, sec. 1, p.18.
48. See *Biur Halakhah, Orah Hayyim* 329 s.v. *ela lefi sha'ah* in which reference is made to the doubts of the *Ba'al Halakhot Ketanot* as to whether or not a seriously injured child may be saved on the Sabbath.
49. *M. Ohol.* 7:6, and see above, notes 27–31.
50. *T. Shab.* 15-7; *Shab.* 135b; *Nidd.* 44b; *Tosafot Shab.* 136a s.v. *mimhal.*
51. R. Isaiah Pik in *Resp. Noda Beyehuda* 2, *Hoshen Mishpat* no. 59; see E. Ellison, 'The foetus in Jewish law' (Heb.), *Sinai* 66 (5730), 39.
52. *id.*
53. *M. Nidd.* 5:3.
54. See the sources cited in n.51 above.
55. *Resp. Noda Beyehuda* 2 *Hoshen Mishpat* no. 59; Ellinson, *op. cit.* p.39. The question of whether or not a full term of nine months is required before the Sabbath can be desecrated for the sake of foetal life is also dealt with by R. Landau in his *responsum.*
56. *Resp. Melamed Leho'il, Yoreh Deah* no. 69; see Ellinson, *op. cit.,* who categorises this view as a weak opinion. However, it is arguable that Ellinson disregards the seriousness of the debate between R. Isaiah Pik and R. Landau on this point *(Resp. Noda Beyehuda* 2 *Hoshen Mishpat* no. 59) and fails to take into account the relevance of non-viability as a factor in determining the question of whether or not the Sabbath may be profaned for the sake of a newly born infant: see also n.62. below.
57. *T. Ter.* 7:20; and see n.4.
58. *Resp. Panim Meirot* 3 no. 8; *Resp. Maharam Shick, Yoreh Deah* no. 155; see Ellinson, op. cit. p.47.
59. *Resp. Mahaneh Hayyim* 2, *Hoshen Mishpat* no. 50.
60. See p.50 above.

61. See end of first section. It is also noteworthy that in the context of foeticide, Maimonides rules that therapeutic abortion is justified on the basis of the aggressor principle, i.e. if A pursued B with the obvious intention of killing him, then A may be stopped even at the cost of his own life. The question that arises is the reason for restricting the preference for maternal life in a situation of conflict to the foetal stage. Surely the pursuer principle would also justify sacrificing a newly born infant for the sake of its mother's life? The general trend in the many attempts to answer this question is based upon an acceptance of the fact that the non-viability of the foetus is the main factor in permitting therapeutic abortion. The pursuer principle is employed by Maimonides in order to emphasise the value of foetal life, even in a situation where the abortion is therapeutic in nature: see p.49 above. In this case, too, it is the non-viability of the foetus which provides the major justification for sacrificing it in a situation of conflict with viable life.

62. *Shulhan Arukh, Orah Hayyim* 330:7; and see the sources cited in notes 39–41.

63. See *Resp. Koah Shor* no. 20; R. David Bleich, *Contemporary Halakhic Problems* (New York, 1977), p.362. Although the emphasis here is on adopting less drastic means in the first instance, the outcome is the same, i.e. indirect means are to be used before directly destroying the foetus.

64. See n.35 above.

65. See *Biur Halakhah, Orah Hayyim* 329 s.v. *ela lefi sha'ah.*

66. *Resp. Migei Haharigah* no. 1. R. Efrati's reasoning proceeds in the main along the lines described with respect to sacrificing the life of a newly born infant in the first part of this section. According to R. Efrati, a person who declines to take human life in these circumstances and is prepared instead to meet a martyr's death is a 'holy person'. For a selection of actual *responsa* arising from the Holocaust experience, see I. Rosenbaum, *The Holocaust and the Halakhah* (New York, 1976).

67. E. Ben-Zimra, 'Halakhic decisions relating to the sanctity of life and martyrdom in the Holocaust period' (Heb.), *Sinai* 80 (5737), 151.

68. *Ibid.,* 162, cf. E. Ben-Zimra, 'Bloodshed by necessity in Jewish and Israeli law' (Heb.), *Shenaton Hamishpat Haivri* 3–4 (5736–7), 117.

69. Also see *Lynch* v. *DPP for N. Ireland* [1975] AER 913; *AG* v. *Whelan* (1934) IR 518; A. Simpson, *Cannibalism and the Common Law* (Penguin, 1986).

70. Simpson, *op. cit.* cites various cases in which shipwrecked mariners ate fellow crew members in order to survive, and they usually chose the victim by the drawing of lots in accordance with the 'custom of the sea'. Apparently, this practice was condoned by the authorities and, hence, in *R.* v. *Dudley and Stephens* itself, there was no attempt to conceal the act of cannibalism. In fact, it would appear that the case was brought partly in order to discourage what was beginning to amount to a widespread practice (see especially chs 5 and 9).

71. The court did, however, ask: 'Is it more necessary to kill him than one of the grown men?' (p.287–8). This question might serve as a basis for arguing that if he had been suffering from a fatal disease, it may very well have been more necessary to kill him. Such an interpretation would, however, involve a radical alteration of the

concept of necessity, and as such, is highly questionable in the context of English criminal law.

72. J. Smith and D. Hogan, *Criminal Law* (London, 1982), p.201; G. Williams, *Textbook of Criminal Law* (London, 1978), p.559; L. Fuller, 'The Speluncean explorers', *Harvard Law Review* 62 (1948–9), 616.

73. P. Glazebrook, The necessity plea in English criminal law', *Crambridge Law Journal* (1972a), 118–9.

74. See K. Barth, *3 Church Dogmatics* (Edinburgh, 1961), p.339; N. St John-Stevas, *The Right to Life* (New York, 1964), p.12; P. Ramsey, 'The morality of abortion', in *Moral Problems: A Collection of Philosophical Essays*, ed. J. Rachels (New York, 1971), p.11.

75. See G. Grisez and R. Shaw, *Beyond the New Morality: The Responsibility of Freedom* (London, 1974), ch. 7; J. Finnis, *Natural Law and Natural Rights* (Oxford, 19801), p.86.

76. See D. Louisell, 'Euthanasia and biathanasia: on dying and killing', in *Death, Dying and Euthanasia*, ed. D. Horan and D. Mall, (Maryland, 1980), p.389; Y. Kamisar, 'Some non-religious views against proposed mercy-killing legislation', in *Death, Dying and Euthanasia*, pp.467, 476, cf. G. Williams, 'Mercy-killing legislation: a rejoinder', in *Death, Dying and Euthanasia*, p.488.

77. The two forms of this princple, i.e. the logical and the empirical, are both discussed in the following section.

78. B. Cardozo, *Law and Literature and Other Essays and Addresses* (New York, 1931), p.113. Although Cardozo's view is not universally accepted amongst learned authors (see n.72) it does, nevertheless, seem to reflect the definitive position of the common law on this issue.

79. *Milhemet Mitzva* 32b s.v. *od heshiv;* see also pp.29, 34 above.

80. See R. Elie Munk in his foreword to R. Immanuel Jakobowitz, *Jewish Medical Ethics* (New York 1975), p.27.

81. D. Callahan, 'Bioethics as a discipline', in *Biomedical Ethics and the Law* (ed. J. Humber and R. Almeder (New York, 1977).

82. See J. Mason and R. McCall Smith, *Law and Medical Ethics* (London, 1983), p.188; cf. Callahan, *id.*

83. A. Dyck, 'Beneficient euthanasia and benemortasia: alternative views of mercy', in *Beneficient Euthanasia,* ed. M. Kohl (New York, 1975), p.124.

84. M. Kohl, 'Voluntary beneficient euthanasia', in *Beneficient Euthanasia,* p.139.

85. I. Leibowitz, *Medicine and the Value of Human Life: Meshin Inaugural Lecture in the History of Medicine* (Heb.), (Tel Aviv, 1977).

86. See M. Fogelman, 'Practical *halakhah* and concealed *halakhah*' (Heb.), *Hatsofeh Lehokhmat Yisrael* 15 (5691), 144.

87. L. Alexander, 'Medical science under dictatorship', *New England Journal of Medicine* 241 (1949); G. Sereni, *Into that Darkness: From Mercy-Killing to Mass Murder* (London, 1974).

88. See Kohl. *op. cit.,* p.137; J. Fletcher, 'Ethics and euthanasia', in *To Live and to Die,* ed. R. Williams (New York, 1973), p.114; cf. L. Dawidowicz, *The War Against the Jews 1933–1945* (New York 1975), p.131, who argues that a combination of the two factors of race and an initially sincere mercy-killing programme provided the stimulus for the death camps.

89. See J. Glover, *Causing Death and Saving Lives* (Penguin, 1982), pp.58, 201.

90. In the context of common law jurisdictions, various jurists have based their opposition to legislation aimed at sanctioning the termination of human life on the wedge principle: see Y. Kamisar, 'Some non-religious views against proposed mercy-killing legislation', in *Death, Dying and Euthanasia* ed. D. Horan and D. Mall (Maryland, 1980), p.467: and D. Louisell, 'Euthanasia and biathanasia; on dying and killing, in *Death, Dying and Euthanasia,* p.389; cf. Glover, *op. cit.* p.164 for an opposing view.

MORALITY, POLICY, AND LAW IN THE *HALAKHAH* RELATING TO THE TREATMENT OF THE CRITICALLY ILL

In general, the category applied by contemporary halakhists to problems involving the critically ill is that of the *goses*. This is the category utilised by the classical codifiers of Jewish law for the purpose of regulating the treatment of the terminally ill,[1] and as such, it is supported by traditional usage. The *goses* category is also attractive from the moral point of view. The distinction between precipitating death and removing an impediment is an intuitively acceptable one in moral terms, and is paralleled in other religious and ethical systems.[2] The situation is rather different with respect to the *terefah* category. Traditionally, the context for its application is the criminal law,[3] not the regulations governing the treatment of the terminally ill. Jewish criminal law, however, has not been applied in practice for centuries, and this fact would understandably militate against its application in contemporary times.[4] In moral terms, the exemption of the killer of a *terefah* from capital punishment is clearly a problematic concept. In order to resolve this problem, modern authorities follow Maimonides in emphasising the fact that such a killer is a shedder of blood and remains liable to divine penalties and extra-legal sanctions. The exemption is, therefore, limited to the death penalty. In all other respects, the murder of a *terefah* is a serious offence.[5] Maimonides's skilful interweaving of criminal law policy and positive *halakhah* ensured that the rule exempting the killer of a *terefah* from capital punishment remained a largely inoperative one in Jewish law. The one exception is the case of choosing between lives, which was discussed in the previous chapter. As a result of this exception, contemporary commentators are prepared to call the *terefah* category into service for the purpose of permitting heart transplants in Jewish law. There is no other case in which the *terefah* category has been released from the constraints of halakhic policy.

In the first section of the present chapter, the apparent superiority of the *goses* model over the *terefah* for the purpose of dealing with the treatment of the critically ill in Jewish law is subjected to critical examination. In the second section, the issue of suffering as a value in this area of the *halakhah* is raised, and the extent to which it might constitute an operative element in a decision to terminate the life of a *terefah* ·is discussed. In this second section, the relationship between *halakhah* and policy in the context of aborting defective foetuses is also analysed. The chapter concludes with a survey of the ramifications of the *terefah* category for the treatment of the critically ill in modern medicine, and a discussion of this category from the broader perspective of the methods by which traditional systems adapt to changing situations.

Critique of the Goses Category

Both the definition of *gesisah* and the distinction between precipi-tating death and removing an impediment in the classical codes of Jewish law are rooted in the concept of natural death.[6] There is clearly a wide gap between this concept and the contemporary situation in which advances in medical science provide the means of keeping alive individuals who have lost almost all their capacity for independent physiological functioning. Modern halakhists, therefore, have modified both the definition of *goses* and the nature of the distinction between precipitation of death and impediment removal in order to overcome this gap. Although there are dissenting views,[7] most halakhists treat *gesisah* as a concept which may be applied independently of its traditional symptons.[8] R. Waldenburg bridges the above-mentioned gap by means of the concept of final-phase *gesisah,* in which all treatment, including nutrituion and respiration, may be terminated.[9] A final-phase *goses* has lost all capacity for basic physiological functioning, and the loss is irreversible. R. Waldenburg argues that in this state, all forms of life-support constitute impediments and may be removed. The real issue has now become the definition of death. In effect, R. Waldenburg has ruled that it is unneccesssary to attempt to resuscitate a clinically dead person. Other authorities distinguish between medical care and basic physiological activities. The latter never constitute impediments and may not be terminated until the establishment of death.[10] Once again, the crucial issue has become the definition of death, and the *goses* category is virtually emptied of all significance for the real problem of the critically ill in modern medicine.

Now, even if it is argued that the conceptual gap between the traditional *goses* and the modern critically ill patient is not an unbridgeable one, the distinction between precipitating death and impediment removal is open to question on purely moral grounds. Distinctions between types of acts in relation to the treatment of the dying are not as popular amongst moral philosophers as they were once. It has, for example, been argued that the 'bare difference between killing and letting die does not, in itself, make a moral difference'.[11] Moreover, marshalling a whole range of arguments in favour of such a distinction is not particularly productive, since 'combining several unpersuasive arguments cannot make a persuasive one'.[12] It has also been suggested that distinctions of this nature are particularly open to abuse and may easily be used in order to cloak activities of a highly immoral nature.[13] In fact, it would appear that to a certain extent the *halakhah* supports this critical view of act distinctions, in this area of the law at least. R. Waldenburg, whose views regarding the *goses* were cited above, reduces the notion of indirectness which is implicit in the classical *goses* category to a purely secondary role. At the end of his *responsum,* he relates to the suggestion made by the director of the hospital requesting the decision that the respirator be disconnected by indirect means only. The specific recommendation was that the machine should be controlled by a time switch. In this way, there would be no direct disconnection of the respirator. R. Waldenburg does not regard this recommendation as mandatory, but observes that it is 'indeed most praiseworthy'. He also takes great pains to emphasise that nothing should be allowed to detract from the major issue, which is the establishment of the irreversible loss of all independent capacity for the vital physical functions. Hence, care must be taken to ensure that there is sufficient time for the patient to be thoroughly examined and his condition determined with a maximum degree of certainty before treatment is discontinued. Clearly, the issue of indirectness is of secondary significance only, the main justification being the establishment of irreversible loss.

The secondary nature of indirectness as a justifying factor in decisions on questions of life and death is supported by the *halakhah* governing both the sacrifice of a *terefah* for the sake of viable life and foeticide. With respect to the *terefah*, it has already been observed that where there is a conflict between the life of a *terefah* and that of a viable or potentially viable individual, that of the latter takes precedence. The main justification for this provision is that the blood of a *terefah* is 'less red' than that of a viable individual. However, the life of a *terefah* may be taken only in an indirect fashion. Indirectness is, therefore, a secondary requirement which comes into operation once the basic justification, i.e. the non-viability of the *terefah,* has been established.[14]

This relationship between viability and the distinction between direct and indirect acts would also appear to be implicit in Maimonides's position regarding the permissibility of therapeutic abortion in Jewish law. Maimonides maintains that the basis for the Mishnaic ruling which permits therapeutic abortion is the pursuer principle,[15] i.e. the foetus is pursuing the mother and threatening her life and, as a result, the foetus may be aborted in the same way that a pursuer may be killed in order to prevent him from murdering his intended victim.[16] One of the various objections to this approach is that there is no reason to limit the scope of the pursuer principle to the stage prior to birth, which is the definitive halakhic position and one which Maimonides himself accepts. In order to rescue Maimonides from this difficulty, one widely accepted tactic is to argue that the pursuer principle is of secondary significance only. The major consideration in permitting therapeutic abortion is, in fact, the pre-natal non-viability of the foetus.[17] The use of the pursuer principle in this context merely adds justificatory force, and serves as a deterrent to unjustified abortion. This explanation of Maimonides's ruling is clearly along the same lines as the explanation adduced in relation to the secondary role played by the formal notion of indirectness in sanctioning the termination of life in the case of the *terefah.* In both instances the physical condition of the individual concerned is the principal justification for sacrificing the life of that individual, and the criterion of indirectness and the pursuer principle enter the picture in a secondary capacity by adding force to the main justification.

On this basis it is arguable that the distinction between types of acts as a primary justificatory criterion in relation to the *goses* is something of an aberration. If it is also recalled that the distinction originated in a medieval pietist tract which was incorporated into the

Shulhan Arukh as part of an Ashkenazic tradition and was often the subject of disapproval by Rabbinic authorities,[18] then this argument is not as unconvincing as it may seem at first glance. It should serve at the very least to raise a question with regard to the superiority of the *goses* over the *terefah* criterion on moral grounds.

The *terefah* category itself, however, is hardly free from moral disadvantages. Nevertheless, upon closer examination, these disadvantages may not be as serious as is commonly supposed. An obvious moral objection to the *terefah* model is that it appears to condone the killing of a perfectly innocent individual who, although suffering from a fatal disease, may still be capable of 'eating, drinking and walking about on the streets'.[19] This objection was met by Maimonides whose invocation of divine and extra-legal penalties takes most of the edge off it. In operative terms, therefore, the shadow of punishment falls upon any person involved in the killing of a *terefah,* even though he or she is legally exempt from the death penalty.[20] This defence to the apparent immorality of the terefah category has been referred to above and need not be repeated here.

A more serious objection is undoubtedly the notion that viability is a legitimate criterion for determining the relative value of human lives in a situation where a choice between them must be made. This notion has been referred to here already; in particular, in the course of the comparative treatment of Jewish and common law regarding the necessity plea in murder cases.[21] It will be recalled that the defence of the halakhic approach in that context was based mainly upon the wide range of divine and extra-legal penalties pending against the legally exempt killer. Since the common law lacks any such institutional devices for protecting social morality, it cannot afford to sanction any active choice between lives. The point of raising the same issue here is to offer a critique of the moral validity of the position adopted by the common law in this type of situation and, hence, to provide a broad moral justification for the halakhic approach.

In effect, the common law adopts a 'hands off' policy in these difficult cases involving choices between lives. There is, nevertheless, some measure of recognition afforded to the moral dilemma engendered by cases of this nature in the form of commuted sentences and pardons for those involved in making such tragic choices (as in the case of a the shipwrecked mariners discussed in the previous chapter). No guidance, however, is provided for dealing with such cases on a priori basis. Jewish law, on the other hand, does provide the means for making such tragic choices in a principled fashion. The relevant criterion is indeed a biological one, but there is nothing immoral about such a criterion. In effect, it is admitted in practice, if not in theory, by the common law itself. The divine and extra-legal sanctions in relation to the *terefah* serve to ensure that any such decision conforms to the spirit as well as to the letter of the *halakhah*. On this view, it is arguable that it is not the *halakhah* but the common law, which ought to be examined in terms of its moral validity. The effect of the common law position is to create a moral vacuum, particularly in a pluralistic society united only by the claims of positive law. In the final analysis, such a vacuum may very well be more dangerous for society than the apparently lower moral standard set by Jewish law in the form of the criterion of viability for choosing between lives. The unsettling effects of this type of moral vacuum are clearly visible in the field of modern bioethics. Although there is a deeply felt social need for some legislation to govern the development and use of scientific advances in modern medicine, the absence of any shared basis for the development of the relevant laws makes any such legislation well nigh unobtainable. At the same time, scientific advances continue to be made almost daily, and the problems that the law sets out to resolve are made only more complex and more pressing by the passage of time.[22]

In moral terms, therefore, the category of *terefah* might very well prove to be more defensible than would at first appear. At least it offers some guidance in cases of conflict between lives, and in relation to matters of life and death it is arguable that some guidance is better than none at all. Serious problems regarding the moral basis for many of the basic notions in relation to questions of life and death in the common law tradition have been raised by moral philosophers. Their argument is that without a clearer understanding of the morality of the law, its provisions are merely sources for confusion.[23] It is this type of charge which the halakhic approach can rebut with facility.

Policy and Law in the Halakhah Relating to the Treatment of the Critically Ill

It is to Maimonides's credit that the rule exempting the killer of a *terefah* from capital punishment became devoid of any significance except in the case of sacrificing a *terefah* for the sake of viable life. As shown in Chapter 3, Maimonides achieved this goal by means of the skilful development of moral principles, divine sanctions, and extra-legal penalties. It was also demonstrated in that chapter that this deployment was entirely consistent with the policy of Jewish criminal law in Talmudic and Midrashic sources. It might be noted in passing that the elaboration of halakhic policy fits in with Maimonides's integrated approach to Jewish law in general. For Maimonides, *halakhah* represents much more than positive law: it also contains the values of Judaism.[24] Maimonides carried out a similar operation with regard to the *halakhah* governing foeticide. This operation was also referred to above,[25] although it was not accomplished in the same elegant fashion as in the context of killing a *terefah*. Maimonides's incorporation of the pursuer principle into the justification for permitting therapeutic abortion did indeed provide a strong basis for protecting foetal life and permitting abortion only in cases involving a direct threat to the life of the mother. At the same time, however, it represents a break with Talmudic tradition, and is subject to internal inconsistencies which remain unresolved to the present day. Indeed, one of the principal modern defenders of Maimonides's formulation was forced to argue that since none of Maimonides's contemporaries saw fit to criticise this ruling, it must have been clear to them and, hence, later commentators are merely lacking in understanding, and this is not a reason for discounting Maimonides's position.[26] Nevertheless, any halakhist wishing to rule leniently on the issue of abortion in Jewish law must either distinguish Maimonides's strict formulation of the *halakhah* on therapeutic abortion or find a way of discounting it.

The question arises now of the strength of halakhic policy of this type in situations where there is a competing moral value at stake. It has already been established that the sacrifice of a *terefah* for the sake of saving a viable life does, in fact, constitute such a case. Since a *terefah* is not viable, his life may be sacrificed for the sake of a viable, or potentially viable, individual. In the context of abortion, an interesting development is the debate which arose between R. Waldenburg and R. Feinstein on the question of aborting a foetus stricken with Tay–Sachs disease.[27] R. Waldenburg argued that this hereditary disease, which causes physical and mental retardation and culminates in certain death by the age of four years, constitutes sufficient grounds for justifying an abortion. According to R. Waldenburg, the major basis for permitting therapeutic abortion in

Jewish law is the fact that a foetus is not considered a living being and, hence, may be sacrificed for the sake of saving maternal life. In the present case, the distress and suffering caused to the mother by the birth and subsequent deterioration of her child, coupled with the suffering undergone by the child itself, were sufficient to justify an abortion. In addition to the basic principle that a foetus is not considered a living being in Jewish law, R. Waldenburg also cited various authorities whose liberal rulings on abortion were based on a wide interpretation of the criterion of maternal life. According to these authorities, this criterion included considerations such as 'great shame'[28] and 'great need'.[29] R. Waldenburg grapples with the Maimonidean position by citing various authorities who deal with the difficulties in Maimonides's formulation by de-emphasising its stricter ramifications and placing it more solidly within the Talmudic tradition according to which the foetus is not a living being and, hence, may be aborted for the sake of preserving maternal life. R. Waldenburg's decision was strongly criticised by R. Feinstein, mainly on the grounds that neither he nor his major precedents attached sufficient weight to Maimonides's strict approach to therapeutic abortion in Jewish law. Also, R. Feinstein cast doubt on the authenticity of two of R. Waldenburg's sources, and dismissed two others on the basis of bibliographical and intellectual incompetence, respectively. R. Feinstein concluded his critique with a strong plea for resisting any attempt at liberalising abortion legislation anywhere in the world. R. Waldenburg came to his own defence, and counter-attacked in relation to both specific criticisms and methodology. With respect to method, R. Waldenburg made the following protest:

> With all great respect, this is not the way things are done. Many scholars have attempted to reconcile conflicting statements . . . in this area, and not one of them suggested that this could be done simply by declaring a printing error![30]

The question of methodology is an important one, and will be taken up in the following section. At present, however, the important point is that R. Waldenburg was prepared to extend the justification for therapeutic abortion to a Tay–Sachs foetus and to emphasise the prevention of suffering as an important element in his decision. Indeed, R. Waldenburg referred to the suffering of both parents as well as the child. He did not limit himself to that of the mother alone.[31] In R. Waldenburg's view, therefore, it is evident that the prevention of suffering in general—and not merely a direct threat to maternal life—is sufficient to overcome the halakhic policy of treating foeticide as a form of bloodshed. Although the issue remains open, it may be concluded that according to R. Waldenburg at least, the possibility of avoiding general suffering made available by techniques for establishing genetic diseases such as Tay–Sachs in foetuses is sufficiently strong to overcome the policy of Jewish criminal law in favour of prohibiting all abortions except those carried out in order to remove a direct threat to maternal life.

To what extent, if any, is the suffering of a critically ill person relevant in Jewish law? The general position regarding the *goses* is that suffering *per se* is not an operative element in permitting the discontinuation of life-supporting treatment. In the words of R. Jehiel Epstein:

> And even though we see that the *goses* is enduring much suffering and it would be better for him to die, we are forbidden to do any act which would precipitate his death.[32]

In this context, however, it is necessary to distinguish between two types of suffering. The first is mainly spiritual in nature, and is caused purely by the soul being prevented from emerging at the proper time.[33] The other is ordinary physical suffering. It would appear that even when Rabbinical authorities do address themselves to the concept of suffering in this area, they do not make it clear whether they are dealing with the first form or the second. Clearly, the former transcends the boundaries of rational determination, and it has indeed been observed that the establishment of the proper time for the soul to leave the body is not a matter which falls within ordinary Rabbinic competence.[34]

In relation to ordinary physical suffering, the practice of praying for the death of a suffering individual, or stopping those praying for his survival from persisting in their devotions, is an accepted one in the *Talmud* and *Midrash*.[35] It is, therefore, permissible to pray for the death of a suffering individual.[36] Contemporary halakhists, however, insist upon a strict separation between this permission and any human action directed towards terminating the life of a terminally ill person.[37] Although Jewish law rejects the notion that suffering must be borne as part of a divinely willed scheme of things,[38] it is not prepared to sanction mercy-killing.

It is noteworthy that in dealing with the issue of suffering as a factor in determining the treatment of the fatally ill, the authorities have addressed themselves solely to the category of *goses,* and not to that of *terefah.* In the light of the above-mentioned decision of R. Waldenburg concerning the abortion of defective foetuses, it is therefore possible to raise the question of whether suffering might constitute a sufficiently strong value to overcome the policy of the *halakhah* regarding the killing of a *terefah.* Is it conceivable that in the same way that R. Waldenburg invoked the suffering of the child as well as that of the mother, in order to overcome halakhic policy against permitting foeticide, the suffering of a *terefah* could provide the justification for terminating his life in an indirect fashion, notwithstanding that no other viable life is at stake? This question must, however, be left open in the hope that it will eventually be addressed by halakhic authorities. R. Waldenburg's *responsum* on the abortion of a Tay–Sachs foetus would seem to indicate that the basic ingredients for dealing with this question are available within the *halakhah.* The direction in which the *halakhah* will proceed is a matter for the halakhic authorities of the future.

Tradition and the Biological Revolution

Halakhic bioethics is one of the most popular fields of research in Jewish law at present. The impetus for this engagement has not only been the growing number of pressing problems in this field but also a general quest for traditional wisdom regarding such problems which touch upon the fundamental moral values of Western society. In rising to the occasion, it is possible that commentators have been too eager to demonstrate the relevance of Jewish law and, hence, have tended to avoid some of the methodological and moral problems raised in the previous chapters. There has been little or no analysis of the traditional categories in the area of the treatment of the critically ill from a conceptual or moral perspective, and, more significantly, the policy elements underlying contemporary halakhic rulings have not been elucidated. This book has attempted to redress that balance, albeit in a rather modest fashion. As far as the specific subject of the critically ill is concerned, the analysis of the *terefah* category into its halakhic and policy elements provided a basis for supporting its application to the critically ill patient of modern medicine. The merit, if any, of this argument is that it preserves meaningful traditional forms rather than emptying them of all content and subordinating them completely to a moral principle, even if that principle is enshrined in halakhic policy.

Without the *terefah* category, the treatment of the critically ill will be regulated only by the *goses* model which, at best, provides a partial solution to the hospitalised individual suffering from an incurable and invariably fatal disease. The above-mentioned debate between R. Waldenburg and R. Feinstein on the issue of aborting a defective foetus is a particularly striking illustration of the use of policy as a means of dealing with a changing reality. R. Feinstein's rejection of traditional sources constitutes a thinly veiled policy argument, the validity of which will be examined shortly. R. Waldenburg's approach is casuistic but traditional. From a purely methodological perspective, it is difficult to justify the approach adopted by R. Feinstein, since it seems to undercut the whole basis of a traditional legal system, namely, reliance on precedent. In the context of the critically ill, therefore, there is a need to release the *terefah* category from its policy constraints in order to cope adequately, i.e. in a traditional fashion, with the modern problem of an individual who is suffering from a painful fatal disease and whose life is being preserved by means of sophisticated technology. Possibly a combination of the two categories would provide a firmer basis for the future development of the *halakhah* in this area than the somewhat emasculated form of the *goses* category with which contemporary halakhists are grappling in order to shape an integrated approach to the problem of the critically ill in Jewish law.

The argument advanced here is that policy ought not to constitute the sole means of providing an answer to an objective situation radically different in nature from that which pertained in the past. This is especially the case when a halakhic solution is available, albeit in the form of a category which has not previously been applied in the context under consideration. The constant application of diverse categories to reality is the life-blood of Jewish law, and the stultification of this process as a result of a moral policy cannot bode well for the future of halakhic development. In this respect, Maimonides's approach is open to criticism. The integrated view of *halakhah* taken by Maimonides tends to inhibit halakhic development in areas in which there is a strong policy element such as the killing of a *terefah*. The effect of this policy is to make traditional categories subservient to a particular moral position which may not be as convincing in a different period. Notwithstanding Maimonides's status as a halakhist, this is a serious defect and may very well have contributed to the fact that his code of Jewish law did not win universal acceptance as the authoritative compilation of *halakhah*. This distinction fell to the *Shulhan Arukh,* which displays a much more traditional style in its approach.[39] It might also be observed that Maimonides adopted a highly untraditional view of the nature of legal reasoning in Jewish law. According to the Maimonidean position, reasoning by analogy is incapable of producing results of an apodictic nature. Hence, legal reasoning, which is almost inevitably analogical, is inherently controversial and disputes are capable of resolution only by means of formal techniques such as majority vote. This view also affected Maimonides's classification of the Divine Commandments, and was subjected to strong criticism by his younger contemporary, Nahmanides, and later Rabbinic authorities. The traditionalist view was that analogical reasoning was perfectly valid within the halakhic system, and the fact that it did not possess the intellectual rigour of the Aristolelian syllogism was irrelevant.[40] In this respect, too, Maimonides's position is an untraditional one.

The issue which must now be tackled is the possibility that the restrictive policy of the *halakhah* regarding all forms of bloodshed is, in fact, endemic to the law in this area. In effect, this is the question of whether or not Jewish law accepts the principle of the sanctity of life, and the answer to this question would appear to be in the negative, i.e. Jewish law does not adopt the notion of sanctity of human life, at least not in its strong form.[41] This notion is, in fact, based upon a theological concept, namely the sacred awe engendered by the very experience of being alive.[42] The idea that human life *per se* is intrinsically sacred would seem to be more suited to certain branches of Christianity than to the Jewish tradition. In the latter system, it is generally accepted that life in itself is not endowed with intrinsic holiness; rather, holiness is a state to be achieved by dint of sustained effort.[43] It is therefore somewhat disconcerting to discover contemporary halakhic authorities and commentators whose views are almost identical to the strong version of the sanctity of life principle. In particular, the methodology adopted by R. Feinstein concerning the question of aborting a Tay–Sachs foetus would appear to constitute a rejection of traditional halakhic methodology in favour of a blanket prohibition on virtually any abortion. R. Feinstein's methodology, which was referred to in the above section, consisted *inter alia* of the rejection of various *responsa* which did not correspond to the strict view of abortion as a form of homicide derived in the main from Maimonides's formulation of the law. In addition to the debatable nature of R. Feinstein's conclusions with regard to the nature of foeticide in Jewish law,[44] his approach would seem to favour a general 'sanctity of life' type of principle over the more traditional case-by-case method of halakhic development. The traditional approach is articulated by R. Elie Munk, who deals with the apparent discrepancies between the *halakhah* on abortion and the treatment of the dying and the a priori positions on these issues adopted by some religious and moral systems. According to R. Munk, these discrepancies arise as a result of the case-by-case approach of Jewish law. Solutions of an a priori nature are not typical of the *halakhah*.[45] This is because there is no principle such as that of the sanctity of life which requires such an a priori position to become institutionalised within the system. A definite connection therefore exists between the type of reasoning used in a particular decision and the issue of whether the *halakhah* accepts an a priori notion of the supreme value of human life. On the basis of the argument presented in the present chapter, it is clear that such a notion is operative only at the level of policy; it is not an absolute value.[46] Competing moral values may override it and, hence, the only possible methodology for juristic development of the *halakhah* is that of the case-by-case method.

In the area of the treatment of the critically ill, there are also halakhists whose views approach a 'sanctity of life' type principle, but whose methodology is more traditional than that of R. Feinstein.[47] As in the case of abortion, it is submitted that the cause of this development is the blurring of the distinction between halakhic policy and a priori principles of an absolute nature. In order to provide a basis for the development of a fruitful halakhic approach to bioethical issues, this distinction must be preserved.

The final point to be made relates to the *terefah* category as a model for dealing with the critically ill. Clearly, much of what has been said in the present chapter is aimed at paving the way for the adoption of this category in the *halakhah* in this field. It is, therefore, noteworthy that one of the central features of the *halakhah* of human *tarfut* is that jurisdiction over those involved in the killing of a *terefah* is not in the hands of regular courts, but of extra-judicial bodes operating on the basis of mainly discretionary principles.[48] In this respect, Jewish law is in line with a significant body of contemporary opinion, according to which cases of this type ought to be dealt with by specialised bodies representing diverse moral and legal perspectives, rather than by regular courts of law.[49] It also accords with the traditional attitude of the English, as opposed to the American judiciary on this matter,[50] although it would appear that the wisdom of the extensive judicial jurisdiction in these matters is also being reconsidered in the USA.[51]

Notes
1. See p.8 above.
2. See E. Keyserlingk, *Sanctity of Life* (Montreal, 1979), ch. 5 for a survey of these systems; cf. R. David Bleich, *Jewish Bioethics*, ed. F. Rosner and D. Bleich (New York, 1979), p.270, who denies any precise parallel with the catholic tradition in this area.
3. See p.22 above.
4. An interesting attempt to bring Jewish criminal law into play in relation to the issue of abortion is R. Jacob Emden's argument that a *mamzer* foetus i.e. one which was conceived in an act of adultery or incest may be aborted, since under the criminal law the mother would be liable to the death penalty, notwithstanding her pregnant condition. Hence, the foetus is notionally dead and may be aborted in order to spare his mother and her family from the great distress of giving birth to a *mamzer* (*Resp. She'elat Yaavez* no. 43). This argument is universally rejected by modern halakhists on the grounds that the provisions of the criminal law are no longer relevant: see *Resp. Ziz Eliezer* 13 no. 102; R. Moses Feinstein, 'On the law concerning the killing of a foetus' (Heb.), in *R. Ezekiel Abramski Memorial Volume,* ed. M. Hirschler (Jerusalem, 5735), 469.
5. *Resp. Iggrot Moshe, Yoreh Deah* no. 36; *Resp. Iggrot Moshe, Hoshen Mishpat* no. 73; *Resp. Bet Avi* 2 no. 153; A. Steinberg, 'Mercy-killing in the light of the *halakhah',* (Heb.), *Sefer Assia* 3, ed. A. Steinberg (Jerusalem, 5743), 432. Also see R. Yissachar Frimer, 'Mercy-killing' (Heb.), *Halakhah Urefuah* 4, ed. M. Hirschler (Jerusalem, 5745), 303, who deals with the inapplicability of the *terefah* category to a non-Jewish patient as well as a Jewish one.
6. See p.10 above.
7. See R. David Bleich, 'Ethico-halakhic considerations in the practice of medicine' *Dine Israel* 7 (1976), 129; and *Jewish Bioethics,* 275, n.2.
8. R. Gedalia Rabinowitz, 'The treatment of the critically ill, the *goses* and the definition of death' (Heb.), *Halakhah Urefuah* 1 (5738), 11; R. Moses Hirschler, 'The obligation to save life' (Heb.), *Halakhah Urefuah* 2 (5741), 35; Steinberg, *op. cit.,* p.454.
9. *Resp. Ziz Eliezer* 13 no. 89 and 14 no. 80; see above p.13.
10. See above p.14.
11. J. Rachels, 'Active and passive euthanasia', *New England Journal of Medicine* 292 (1975), 79. Also see I. Kennedy, 'Switching off life support machines: the legal implications', *Criminal Law Journal [1977], 443; G. Williams, 'Euthanasia', Medico-Legal Journal* 14 (1973), 14.

12. R. Veatch, *Death, Dying and the Biological Revolution* (New Haven, 1976) p.93.

13. J. Glover, *Causing Death and Saving Lives* (Penguin, 1982), pp.109, 112; J. Harris, *Violence and Responsibility* (London, 1980), ch. 4.

14. See p.50 above. The notion of indirectness was employed in order to reconcile R. Ezekiel Landau's objection that the direct killing of a *terefah* for the sake of a viable life was 'unheard of', with the view of R. Meiri that it was permitted. From the rhetorical form of R. Landau's objection, it may be inferred that its thrust is moral rather than strictly legal, and the inclusion of the indirectness requirement may therefore be regarded as a moral safeguard in a situation in which the life concerned is forfeit on the grounds of non-viability.

15. *Hil. Rozeah* 1:9.

16. The issue of intention is also a widely discussed problem in Maimonides's formulation of this law. The foetus does not have any intent to kill its mother, whereas an ordinary pursuer does intend the death of the person being pursued. Indeed, this is the basis for the *Talmud's* rejection of the pursuer principle in this context: 'She [the mother] is being pursued by Heaven' *(Sanh.* 72b, and see ch. 3 p. 67 n.61). One solution to this problem is that Maimonides distinguishes between the two senses of the pursuer, one with intent, and the other without. It is in the latter sense that he uses the pursuer principle in the context of therapeutic abortion (see *Hil. Hovel Umazik* 8:25; *Resp. Torat Hesed, Even Haezer* no. 42; A. Enker, *Hekhrah Vezorekh Bedinei Onshin* (Bar Ilan, 5733), 221 n.44; I. Warhaftig, 'Self defence in the crimes of homicide and assault' (Heb.), *Sinai* 81 (5737), 45. This objection is also overcome in the light of the general argument that Maimonides does not mean to displace but merely to complement the main justification for therapeutic abortion, i.e. the non-personhood of the foetus.

17. See p.52 above.

18. See p.11 above.

19. Maimonides, *Hil. Rozeah* 2:8.

20. The spectre of 'possible criminal liability' hovering over 'the path toward decision for withholding treatment' in the case of anomalous newly born babies is approved as a necessary safeguard in this highly controversial area by R. Burt 'Authorizing death for anomalous newborns', *Genetics and the Law,* ed. A. Milansky and G. Annas, (New York, 1975), p.43.

21. See p.57 above.

22. See D. Callahan, 'Bioethics as a discipline', in *Biomedical Ethics and the Law,* ed. J. Humber and A. Almeder, (New York 1977).

23. See Glover, *op. cit.,* ch. 20 on the virtue of 'moral distance' in questions of life and death.

24. See I. Twersky, *Introduction to the Code of Maimonides* (New Haven, 1980), ch. 6.

25. See p.29 above.

26. Feinstein, *op. cit.,* p.463.

27. The debate is in *Resp. Ziz Eliezer* 13 no. 89 and 14 no. 80; Feinstein, *ibid.,* 461–9. For a point-by-point analysis see Appendix A.

28. *Resp. Rav Paalim, Even Haezer* no. 4.

29. *Resp. She'elat Ya'avez* no. 43.
30. *Resp. Ziz Eliezer* 14 no. 80.
31. *Resp. Ziz Eliezer* 13 no. 89.
32. *Arukh Hashulhan, Yoreh Deah* 339:1.
33. See *Sefer Hasidim* no. 234.
34. *Resp. Hatam Sofer, Orah Hayyim* 199; *Resp. Ziz Eliezer* 14 no. 81; Steinberg, *op. cit.* p.454.
35. See *Ket.* 104a; *Tan.* 23a; *Yeb.* 79a; *B.M.* 84a; *Yalkut Shimoni, Ekev* no. 471 and *Prov.* no. 543.
36. R. Nissim Gerondi, commenting on the Talmudic passage which discusses the duty to visit the sick and pray for their recovery *(Ned.* 50a) states that there are times when a man should ask for divine mercy for a suffering individual, that he may die; see also *Ha'amek She'elah, Lev.* 93; *Tiferet Yisrael, Yom.* 8:7; *Arukh Hashulhan, Yoreh Deah* 735:2. According to R. Hayyim Palaggi, such a prayer ought only to be recited by a person who has no direct relationship with the suffering individual concerned *(Resp. Hikkrei Lev* 1 no. 60).
37. See *Resp. Iggrot Moshe, Hoshen Mishpat* no. 73; R. Judah Gershuni, *Kol Zafayikh* (Jerusalem, 5740), 335. This distinction between prayer and action is also reflected in the Talmudic account of the martyrdom of R. Hanina b. Teradyon *(A. Zar.* 18a). According to the *Talmud,* R. Hanina uttered the words: 'Let He who gave me my soul take it away.' He was not, however, prepared to open his mouth so that 'the flames could enter his body', thereby terminating his agony. Undoubtedly, the reason for the apparent divergence between R. Hanina's words and deeds is that prayer and action are not the same, and whereas the former is always permitted, the latter is not.
38. *Resp. Ziz Eliezer* 13 no. 89.
39. See Introduction, p.6.
40. Maimonides emphasises the non-apodictic nature of analogical reasoning both in his *Introduction to the Mishnah,* ed. Y. Kafach (Jerusalem, 1964), p.3 and his *Book of the Commandments,* ed. H. Chavel (Jerusalem, 1981), p.29. Legal syllogisms are expressly excluded from his early work (I. Efros, 'Maimonides' treatise on logic', *Proceedings of the American Academy for Jewish Research* 8 [1937-8]). His belief that all disputes over legal interpretation are only resolvable in a formal fashion is reiterated in various places in his halakhic writings *(Introduction to the Mishnah, id.; Hil. Melakhim,* chs. 1-2). Maimonides's position is strongly criticised by Nahmanides in his glosses on the *Book of the Commandments (ibid.,* 51) and by R. Yair Bachrach in his *Resp. Havot Yair,* no. 192. Also see: J. Blidstein, 'Transmission and institutional authority in the concept of the oral law in Maimonidean thought' (Heb.), *Da'at* 16 (1986), 15.
41. See Keyserlingk, *op. cit.,* ch. 1 for a general survey of this principle and the various forms it takes in religious and moral thought. Also see D. Callahan, 'The sanctity of life', in *Updating Life and Death,* ed. D. Culter (Boston, 1968), p.185 for a critical comment on this principle.
42. See K. Barth, *Church Dogmatics* 3 (Edinburgh, 1961), p.339.

43. See *Encyclopaedia Judaica* 10, p.866.
44. See D. Sinclair, 'The legal basis for the prohibition on abortion in Jewish law', *Israel Law Review* 15 (1980), 126, where the similarity between this approach and the catholic position on abortion is also discussed.
45. R. Elie Munk, foreword to R. Immanuel Jakobowitz, *Jewish Medical Ethics* (New York, 1975), p.27.
46. Cf. I. Leibowitz, *Medicine and the Value of Human Life: Meshin Inaugural Lecture in the History of Medicine* (Heb.), (Tel Aviv, 1977), according to whom this is the position of Jewish tradition and *halakhot* which deviate from it are in the category of those laws which ought to be kept concealed (see p.61 above).
47. See e.g. Bleich, *Jewish Bioethics, op. cit.* p. 275; Y. Levi, 'An impediment to the emergence of the soul' (Heb.), *Noam* 16 (5733), 53. Also see *Resp. Nezer Matai* no. 30.
48. See p.63 above.
49. The issue of the role of the judiciary was raised in relation to the competence of the judges to decide on complex medical matters by the debate following the decision of the Massachusetts Supreme Court in the case of *Superintendent of Belchertown State School* v. *Saikewicz* (1977) 373 Mass. 728, 370 NE 2d. 417. In this decision, the court attempted to define the criteria which judges should use to determine the issue of the quality of life. The decision was sharply attacked by the medical profession, and the ensuing debate illustrates the difficulties involved in attempting to establish formal guidelines for the use of judicial bodies in this area: see W. Curran, 'The Saikewicz decision', *New England Journal of Medicine* 270 (1978), 500; A. Relman, 'The Saikewicz decision: judges as physicians', *New England Journal of Medicine* 270 (1978), 509; cf. C. Baron 'Meical paternalism and the rule of law', *American Journal of Law and Medicine* 4 (1979), 337; also see D. Meyers, *Medico-Legal Implications of Death and Dying* (New York, 1981), p.278; Keyserlingk, *op. cit.,* ch. 8.
50. See J. Mason and R. McCall Smith, *Law and Medical Ethics* (London, 1983), p.189.
51. Mason and McCall Smith, *id.* The American case law is rich in principles and directives for the termination of life-saving treatment: see D. Meyers, *Medico-Legal Implications of Death and Dying* (New York, 1981), p.379. These include the principle enunciated in *Re Quinlan* (1976) 70 NJ 355 A 2d 651 that where there is no medical likelihood that a patient in a long-term coma will return to a conscious, cognitive state with continued life-support therapy, there should be no legal obligation to continue such therapy. In *Re Dinnerstein* (1978) 380 NE 2d 134, it was held that where the patient is not in a persistent vegetative state, but is suffering from an incurable disease as a result of which death is imminent, and continued life-support treatment will only briefly prolong the process of dying, then such treatment may be withdrawn. There are, however, no clear guidelines as to whether 'care', such as nourishment and hygiene may also be withdrawn when medical treatment such as artifical respiration is terminated. Much emphasis is also placed on the wishes of the patient or his family and the opinions of independent physicians. In this context, it is noteworthy that several

decisions have emphasised the need for ethics committees, which would consider diagnosis in difficult cases. In this respect, at any rate, it is apparent that in the USA, too, the need to remove decisions in this area from the formal court setting to a more informal one is recognised and appreciated.

CONCLUSION

Two different modes of reasoning in relation to the bioethical issues discussed in the previous chapters emerge from the present study. The first, which may be termed the Maimonidean mode, is based upon the rational principle of the fundamental importance of human life. This principle is treated as a meta-principle in Jewish law and is used to fill in gaps in the existing *halakhah*. Examples of such gap-filling are the elucidation of a prohibition on non-therapeutic foeticide and the invocation of divine and extra-legal penalties in the case of the killing of a *terefah*. There are, however, aspects of the *halakhah* which are not consistent with this principle, e.g. the statement of *Tosafot* that it is permitted to kill a foetus, and the view according to which a *terefah* may be sacrificed for the sake of a viable life. At the level of principle, too, it is not altogether clear that there are not other, more coherent, candidates for the role of meta-principle in this area. One such candidate is the relationship between diminished viability and sanction discussed at length in Chapter 3. Although one modern thinker has indeed suggested that aspects of *halakhah* which are incoherent or inconsistent with the principle of the fundamental value of every single human life ought to be relegated to the realm of '*halakhah* which is not revealed'[1] most modern authorities who adopt the Maimonidean mode do not need to take such drastic steps in order to preserve their meta-principle in the context of the *halakhah*. In the course of the preceding chapters, there are sufficient examples of the reconciliation of such inconsistencies with the principle of the paramount value of each and every human life, irrespective of its viability, to demonstrate the compelling power of the Maimonidean model even though its application may occasionally require the dismissal of halakhic sources on the grounds of forgery or the incompetence of the learned authors.[2] It was suggested above that the key to the Maimonidean position lay in its moral strength, particularly on the level of social policy. The question that then arises is its continued attractiveness in an area of rapidly shifting moral perceptions. This question will be taken up shortly.

The other mode of reasoning exposed above might be described as the standard mode, and it is characterised by its attempt to discover the most coherent principle in any area of *halakhah*[3] as opposed to a meta-principle drawn, at least in this case, from an external, rational source. In the context of therapeutic abortion, this mode is followed by those authorities who adopt a wide-ranging criterion for maternal welfare and do not rely solely upon Maimonides's strict position based upon a direct threat to maternal life. These authorities maintain that the coherent principle in this area of the *halakhah*—including Maimonides's own complex formulation regarding therapeutic abortion in Jewish law—is that the foetus is not considered a living person for the purposes of the criminal law. A similar result is achieved with respect to the treatment of the critically ill. Here, too, the coherent principle is that diminished viability is a relevant factor when it comes to choosing between lives.

It is arguable that more is at stake here than the question of the extent to which moral policy ought to be incorporated into the body of the *halakhah*. The Maimonidean mode may very well constitute a sceptical position with regard to the process of legal reasoning in general. Certainly, there is ample evidence to suggest that Maimonides himself held such a sceptical view of reasoning in the field of legal argumentation. According to Maimonides, the analogical type of reasoning employed in the juristic development of the *halakhah* is inherently controversial and, hence, scriptural status is denied to all derived law.[4] Maimonides also excluded 'legal syllogisms' from his early work on logical terms,[5] and may very well have been influenced in this respect by classical Islamic jurisprudence.[6] For Maimonides, therefore, rational principles play a particularly important role in the *halakhah,* since there is nothing inherently compelling in the reasoned conclusions of halakhic debates, provided, of course, that such principles do not conflict directly with existing halakhic norms.[7] For Maimonides, it would appear that institutional authority[8] replaced the notion of textual interpretation as the criterion for normative *halakhah*.[9] The extent to which this view of legal argumentation is shared by later authorities is debatable, but it is certainly present in an unarticulated form in several of the *responsa* on foeticide and killing a *terefah* written by authorities following the Maimonidean principle concerning the almost absolute value of human life.

In terms of the reasoning issue, it ought to be noted that Maimonides's view was widely criticised. Nahmanides raised numerous objections to Maimonides's narrow definition of scriptural law, most of which are aimed at demonstrating that the Sages of the *Talmud* did, in fact, include derived laws in the category of scriptural law. According to Nahmanides, all derived laws are scriptural unless there is an exlicit Talmudic statement to the effect that the derivation is merely a literary flourish.[10] Nahmanides's position is echoed by later authorities, all of whom agree that the non-apodictic nature of legal reasoning does not render its conclusions rationally or legally defective.[11] It should also be observed that Maimonides was unique in the interest he took in developing the halakhic infrastructure for judicial, legislative, and executive bodies in Jewish law. Clearly, other halakhists who did not develop, nor see the need for developing, such an infrastructure could not share Maimonides's sceptical approach to legal reasoning.

The standard mode is obviously closer to the traditional approach to legal reasoning adopted by the majority of halakhic authorities throughout the ages. The best illustration of the difference between the Maimonidean and standard modes of reasoning in this area of *halakhah* is undoubtedly the Tay–Sachs foetus debate, which is analysed step-by-step in Appendix A. It is precisely the issue of modes of reasoning which underlies this debate, and it is noteworthy that an issue which is rarely articulated in halakhic sources is so strongly contested in this case. The fact that it is the reasoning issue which takes pride of place in this debate surely bears out the contention made above that the tension between the Maimonidean and standard forms of reasoning constitutes one of the most important elements in contemporary halakhic bioethics.

Throughout the book, the point has been made that, in practice, it is the Maimonidean mode which has been adopted by the majority of modern authorities. It has also been argued that the main reason for this is the moral attractiveness of the Maimonidean position.

Whether or not this position is still as morally attractive as it was is, however, a serious question. Contemporary moral philosophers have criticised the strict view that viability is an irrelevant factor in choosing between lives. Indeed, it has been argued that there is more moral integrity in recognising viability as a factor in such situations than in refusing to do so. Also, this is an area in which moral perceptions are in a process of flux, and it is difficult to predict the form such perceptions will take, even in the near future. From the perspective of the moral image of the *halakhah,* therefore, it may be an opportune time to reconsider the issue of methodology in halakhic bioethics and the possible adoption of a standard type mode of reasoning in this area of Jewish law.

The ramifications of this type of approach for the treatment of the critically ill patient were spelled out in Chapter 4. As a result of the analysis in that chapter, a possible justification was offered for permitting the termination of the life of a critically ill patient who was undergoing great suffering. Support was also found for the use of potential viability as a criterion for allocating scarce medical resources and transplanting vital organs. On the basis of some aspects of contemporary halakhic writings, it is arguable that this approach is becoming more acceptable in halakhic circles and that the halakhic position regarding the critically ill patient may very well develop along the lines mentioned above.

According to the approach based upon the fully-fledged Maimonidean model, however, only a non-physiological impediment to death may be removed from a dying patient. Moreover, the definition of dying is a narrow one answering only to the classical *goses* of halakhic literature. Both the Maimonidean approach and the standard mode are valid halakhic responses to the problem posed by the existence of a twilight zone between life and death created by modern technology. No matter which of the views shapes the future response of Jewish law to this problem, it ought to be abundantly clear that Jewish law possesses a rich and significant body of learning for dealing with it. Tradition, we may conclude, thus displays great potential as an effective way of dealing with the biological revolution.

Notes
1. I. Leibowitz, *Medicine and the Value of Human Life: Meshin Inaugural Lecture in the History of Medicine* (Heb.), (Tel Aviv, 1977); and see p.61 above. Indeed, Leibowitz derives the principle of the absolute value of human life from Maimonidean sources albeit in the area of philosophy rather than *halakhah.*

2. See the Appendix A for a striking illustration of this approach in the context of this debate.

3. See N. MacCormick, *Legal Reasoning and Legal Theory* (Oxford, 1978), to which I am indebted for the usage of the terms 'consistency' and 'coherence' in the context of legal reasoning.

4. *Introduction to the Mishnah,* ed. Y. Kafach (Jerusalem, 1964), p.3; and the *Book of the Commandments,* ed. H. Chavel (Jerusalem, 1981), p.29.

5. See I. Efros, 'Maimonides' treatise on logic', *Proceedings of the American Academy for Jewish Research* 8 (1937–8), 47.

6. See R. Brunschvig, 'Logic and law in classical islam', in *Logic in Classical Islamic Culture,* ed. G. von Grunebaum (Wiesbaden, 1970), p.16.

7. See I. Twersky, *Introduction to the Code of Maimonides* (New Haven, 1980), ch. 6.

8. See J. Blidstein, 'Transmission and institutional authority in the concept of the oral law in Maimonidean thought', (Heb.), *Da'at* 16 (1986), 26.

9. In *Hil. Mamrim* 1:1, Maimonides observes quite forcefully that 'the great Court in Jerusalem is the mainstay of the Oral law'.

10. *Book of the Commandments, ibid.* 51.

11. See Ritva, *Rosh Hashanah* 16a, *s.v. umalkhuyot; Resp. Havot Yair* no. 162.

APPENDIX A
THE TAY-SACHS FOETUS DEBATE

According to R. Eliezer Waldenburg, the abortion of a foetus suffering from Tay-Sachs disease[1] is permitted until the seventh month of pregnancy. Although this time limit is an innovation, the decision was based upon a number of precedents as well as upon the generally accepted view that abortion is not a form of homicide in Jewish law. The principal precedent was a *responsum* of R. Jacob Emden,[2] according to whom an abortion may be performed in a case of 'great need', i.e. where the foetus is harming the mother, even if her life is not in danger. R. Waldenburg ruled that this was a classic case for the application of this criterion in the light of the tragic results of the birth for both parents and child. The fact that the suffering involved may be of a mental rather than a physical nature does not detract from the 'great need' of this case since mental distress is often more severe than physical pain.

In R. Moses Feinstein's view, however, it is forbidden to abort a Tay–Sachs foetus, since there is no prima-facie threat to the mother's life. Neither great suffering nor parental sickness override the prohibition on abortion, which constitutes a form of homicide. Thus, R. Feinstein recommends observant doctors to refrain from testing for Tay–Sachs disease, since they would feel constrained from performing an abortion and would therefore only increase the suffering of the parents; alternatively, they would be responsible for the abortion being performed by a non-observant physician.

R. Feinstein's decision is based on the following arguments:
- a. According to *Tosafot*,[3] abortion is forbidden to Jews on the basis of the rule that 'there is nothing permitted to Jews which is forbidden to Noahides'.[4] Since R. Yishmael teaches that

abortion is a capital crime under Noahide law,[5] it follows that it must be prohibited for Jews. Although *Tosafot* do not explain the nature of this prohibition, R. Feinstein argues that it is a prohibition of homicide.

b. In tractate *Niddah, Tosafot* state that although it is permitted to kill a foetus, the Sabbath may still be profaned in order to save its life.[6] According to R. Feinstein, 'it is absolutely clear that we are dealing with a scribal error and the text ought to read *patur* (exempt) instead of *mutar* (permitted)'. The *Tosafot* would then read: 'Although one is exempt from punishment for killing the foetus, one is still . . . ' etc. All that can then be inferred from this *Tosafot* is the possibility that the prohibition on abortion is not accompanied by any legal sanction.

c. It is generally accepted that the Sabbath may be profaned in order to save foetal life.[7] This would not be the case unless abortion was considered homicide for no such dispensation would be granted unless foetal life was protected by the *halakhah* on a normative basis. R. Feinstein also criticises the view, attributed to Nahmanides, that such dispensation is granted even though abortion is not homicide.

d. Maimonides invokes the principle of *rodef,* according to which it is mandatory to take the life of a pursuer in order to save his victim,[8] in formulating the Mishnaic ruling[9] that the mother's life takes precedence over that of the foetus.[10] By doing so, he implies that the foetus is a life (and abortion a form of homicide), for why else would he have recourse to a justificatory principle normally applied to the killing of fully viable human beings?

Many authorities take the view that Maimonides's use of the pursuer principle is merely a means of qualifying the main Talmudic proposition that as long as the foetus has not emerged into the light of the world, it is not a human life.[11] It does not make the foetus into a full human being.

R. Feinstein is severely critical of these views: 'It is sheer vanity to maintain that Maimonides' language is not precise; such a charge constitutes a general libel on all his works . : . earlier and greater scholars did not question this point, for they realised that Maimonides would be able to resolve any difficulty.' R. Feinstein resolves Maimonides's formulation in his own fashion, preserving the implication that abortion constitutes homicide.[12]

e. According to R. Jair Bachrach,[13] the foetus is a person for purposes of the law of homicide only after the onset of labour. R. Feinstein dismisses this distinction, since it is based on the *Tosafot* cited in *(b)* above, which he rejected on the grounds of scribal error.

f. In the view of R. Joseph Trani, abortion is permitted even where there is no danger to maternal life.[14] R. Feinstein points out that R. Trani's responsa are contradictory, for in one case he gives a lenient ruling and in another his ruling is more restrictive. Moreover, in his lenient ruling R. Trani does not mention Maimonides's opinion and, therefore, 'this *responsum* is to be ignored, for it is undoubtedly a forgery, compiled by an errant disciple and falsely ascribed to him'.

   Further evidence of this forgery may be deduced from the precedent cited in the *responsum* to the effect that Nahmanides assisted a non-Jewish woman to abort her foetus. The source for this account is given as a *responsum* of Rashba, but in fact no such *responsum* exists. Moreover, if it were authenticated, the precedent would be confined to the first forty days of pregnancy, in accordance with Nahmanides's views, as applied to Noahides.[15]

g. R. Feinstein criticises a lenient decision of R. Joseph Hayyim on the grounds that he only adverts to one of R. Joseph Trani's two *responsa,* and that he seems to imply that he did not have a sufficient library at his disposal while writing the *responsum.*[16]

h. One of the leading permissive *responsa* in this area is that of R. Jacob Emden allowing the abortion of a *mamzer* (bastard) foetus.[17] R. Feinstein criticises the somewhat bizarre reasoning in the first part of the decision, and consequently rejects the whole *responsum.*

In R. Feinstein's view, there was no basis for R. Waldenburg's decision that a Tay–Sachs foetus could be aborted until seven months. R. Waldenburg relied on precedents which were either forged or simply wrong, and no reliance whatsoever may be placed on the decision. R. Feinstein also observed that the very phrase upon which R. Waldenburg placed so much emphasis (i.e. the 'great need' class) meant, when properly understood, that abortions ought *not* to be performed in such instances!

R. Waldenburg came to his own defence, and counter-attacked both in terms of general methodology and specific criticisms. In the course of his argument, R. Feinstein had dismissed two offending sources (Tosafot, R. Joseph Trani) as forgeries, and two more (R. Joseph Hayyim, R. Jacob Emden) on other grounds. In R. Waldenburg's words:

> With all great respect, this is not the way things are done. Many scholars attempted to reconcile conflicting statements of the Tosafot in this area, and not one of them suggested that this could be done simply by declaring a printing error!

It is unusual for a halakhic dispute to be resolved by declaring inconvenient sources to be forgeries, and the employment of such tactics raises doubts as to the legal integrity of the argument as a whole. (In any case, R. Feinstein's own remarks are a sufficient indication of this strong concern for the decline in moral standards following in the wake of liberal abortion legislation, and it is therefore more than likely that it is this concern which is the operative factor in his analysis of the law).

In answer to specific criticisms, R. Waldenburg points out that:

a There is no general consensus as to the nature of the prohibition stated by Tosafot. Many authorities maintain that it is merely Rabbinical,[18] and others that it is unknown.[19] The search for the legal basis for the prohibition is, moreover, the one consistent theme in almost every treatment of this topic from the Middle Ages down to the present day.

b Many authorities explain the statement of the Tosafot in niddah in different terms,[20] or take it at its face value and maintain that it reflects the view of the tana kama who disagrees with R. Yishmael's opinion that foeticide is a capital crime under Noahide law.[21]

c R. Waldenburg does not accept the causal link between dispensation to save foetal life on the Sabbath and the law of abortion. Citing various authorities, he argues that the issues are to be treated separately, and relies upon Nahmanides's view to explain that the dispensation is based on the future potential of the foetus to observe many Sabbaths, rather than relating to its present status.[22]

d Numerous authorities explain Maimonides's ruling without concluding that the foetus is a person and that abortion is homicide.[23] R. Feinstein's contention that the problematic aspect of Maimonides's formulation was not raised until recently is inaccurate, and his own argument is circular. Furthermore, it is a moot point whether Maimonides himself held that nothing is forbidden to a Noahide but permitted to a Jew.[24]

e With respect to R. Joseph Trani's *responsa,* it is possible to reconcile them both in a satisfactory manner without declaring them to be the work of an indefatigable forger.[25] Evidence of the authenticity of both *responsa* may be culled from the fact that one of his main disciples, R. Hayyim Benveniste, cited both of them in his glosses to the *Shulhan Arukh.*[26]

The inclusion in the account of Nahmanides having assisted a non-Jewish woman in aborting her foetus in R. Trani's *responsum* is not conclusive evidence of forgery of that *responsum,* since the Rashba did, in fact, give such an account in his collection of *responsa (Resp. Rashba* 1, no. 120) but the context in which it was applied by R. Trani was misunderstood both by R. Feinstein and by others.[27] Rashba states that Nahmanides rendered paid medical assistance to a non-Jewish woman in childbirth, but does not mention abortion. It is R. Trani who goes on to explain that assisting in an abortion would also be permitted. The link with abortion is made by R. Trani in the form of an extrapolation from the *responsum* dealing with medical assistance at childbirth!

f R. Feinstein's negative view of R. Joseph Hayyim's *responsum* is not entirely justified in the light of a careful reading of the text. R. Hayyim does mention both *responsa* of R. Trani, but he chooses to rely on the more lenient one. Nowhere does he indicate a shortage of books or that he is writing without access to works of reference, and there is therefore no reason to dismiss the *responsum* on these grounds.

g R. Jacob Emden's distinction between a regular foetus and a *mamzer* one is unacceptable. His criterion of 'great need', however, is a separate ground, and as such constitutes a valid precedent. R. Feinstein's contention that the phrase used by R. Emden in qualifying the application of this criterion, i.e. 'there is a ground for arriving at a lenient decision', means that there are many more grounds for not doing so, is far-fetched. In the light of all this, R. Waldenburg concludes: 'Our view remains unchanged and abortion is permitted in a case of a Tay–Sachs foetus until seven months.'

Notes

1. This disease is a hereditary condition prevalent amongst babies born to Jews of East European origin. It causes physical and mental retardation, loss of sight and hearing and death by the age of three or four years.
2. *Resp. She'elat Yaavetz* no. 43.
3. *Sanh.* 59a, s.v. *leka; Hull.* 33a, s.v. *ehad.*
4. *Sanh.* 59a.
5. *Sanh.* 57b.
6. *Nidd.* 44a, s.v. *ihu.*
7. *Arak.* 7b.
8. *Sanh.* 72b.
9. *M. Ohol.* 7:6.
10. *Hil. Rozeah* 1:9.
11. *Resp. Noda Beyehuda* 2, *Hoshen Mishpat* 59; *Resp. Koah Shor* no. 20; *Resp. Torat Hesed* no. 42.
12. 'Diagnosis of foetal health and the prohibition of abortion', *Halakhah and Medicine* 1 (1980), 304.
13. *Resp. Havot Yair* no. 31.
14. *Resp. Maharit* nos. 97, 99.
15. *Novallae* on *Nidd.* 44b; *Torat Ha'adam, inyan hasakanah s.v. uvehilkhot.*
16. *Resp. Rav Pa'alim, Even Haezer* no. 4.
17. *She'elat Yaavetz* no. 43.
18. e.g. R. Samuel Kaidanower, *Resp. Emunat Shemu'el;* R. Schneour Zalman of Lublin, *Resp. Torat Hesed* no. 31; R. Solomon Kluger, *Resp. Hayyim Veshalom* 1 no. 40, and see *Sede Hemed, Kelalim Ma'arekhet Ha'alef* 19, 1, 304.
19. R. Yehiel Weinberg, *Resp. Seridei Esh* 3 no. 127.
20. R. Joseph Rosen, *Resp. Zofnaṭ Paneah* 1 no. 59; R. Eliezer Waldenburg, *Resp. Ziz Eliezer* 9 no. 51.
21. *Torat Hesed,* no. 31; R. Hayyim Ozer Grodzinski, *Resp. Ahiezer* 3 no. 65.
22. *Ziz Eliezer* 9 no. 51.
23. Sema, *Hoshen Mishpet* 425:8; R. David b. Zimra, *Resp. Radbaz* 2 no. 695; *Torat Hesed* no. 31; *Ziz Eliezer* 9 no. 51.
24. R. Moses Sofer, *Resp. Hatam Sofer, Yoreh Deah* 19; R. Samuel Engel, *Resp. Maharash Engel* 5 no. 89.
25. *Ziz Eliezer* 9 no. 51.
26. *Sheeirei Knesset Hagedolah, Yoreh Deah* 154.
27. R. Isser Unterman, 'Regarding the obligation to save the life of a foetus', (Heb.) *Noam* 6 (1963), 9.

APPENDIX B
THE GENERAL POSITION REGARDING THE
TERMINATION OF THE LIFE OF A
CRITICALLY ILL PATIENT IN
ANGLO-AMERICAN LAW

The general position in English law is that 'mercy-killing' is no different from murder.[1] It would, however, appear that if a doctor can show that the particular life-shortening treatment administered to a patient was intended primarily to relieve pain and not to kill, then he will almost certainly be acquitted of a charge of murder. According to an *obiter dictum* of J. Devlin in *R. v. Adams,*[2] 'The doctor is entitled to relieve pain and suffering even if the measures he takes may incidentally shorten life.' The test is, in fact, the 'double-effect' doctrine developed by the Catholic Schoolmen and accepted by the Church of England.[3] The idea of double effect was relied upon in the relatively recent case of *R. v. Arthur*[4] in which a paediatrician was charged with the murder of a Down's syndrome baby in whose treatment notes he had written: 'Parents do not wish it to survive. Nursing care only.' The baby died about three days later. During the course of the trial, the charge was reduced to one of attempted murder, and in his direction to the jury, J. Farquharson observed that a conclusion to the effect that 'eminent doctors have evolved standards that amount to committing a crime' ought to be reached only after long and hard thought on the matter. Dr Arthur was acquitted of attempted murder.

In the light of these cases, the contemporary position regarding 'mercy-killing' in England has been summarised as follows:

> no British jury is likely to adjudge a doctor guilty of a serious offence when applying the principle of double effect in good faith. Prosecution is now extremely unlikely in such circumstances.[5]

There is, however, no clear basis for the double-effect principle in the common law tradition. Although it has been argued that the decision in R. v. Adams can be explained in terms of the defence of necessity,[6] it was demonstrated in chapter 4 that this is not the generally accepted view in the common law. Indeed, it was observed by Lord Edmund Davies that 'killing both pain and patient may be good morals but it is far from certain that it is good law'.[7]

In the final analysis, therefore, the lesson to be learned from the cases in this area would seem to be practical rather than doctrinal. Thus far, it would appear that English law has avoided the American trend towards the direct involvement of the courts in the problems of treating the critically ill. There are no 'allowing to die' statutes along the lines of the California Natural Death Act, 1976, and no clear precedents on the criminal implications of disconnecting a respirator from a critically ill patient. It is nevertheless clear that the termination of artificial respiration on the grounds that the patient is dead does not break the chain of causation in the criminal law.[8] In general, the judges are inclined to rely upon good medical practice, and leave decisions in relation to what they obviously regard as clinical and ethical judgements to doctors and those closely concerned with the patient in question. Indeed, it has been suggested that the American trend, with its activist approach to the problems of the critically ill and the dying, has brought about a situation in which confusion about the law has resulted in the practice of 'defensive medicine' with respect to the critically ill.[9]

The issue of whether or not switching off an artificial respirator constitutes the crime of murder has been discussed by learned writers.[10] No definitive conclusion would seem to have been reached and, once again, it is pointed out that the typical jury in a criminal trial would probably distinguish between a well-wisher disconnecting a respirator and the same step taken by a doctor. In this context, too, the general conclusion would appear to be that 'the great majority of life or death decisions can be based on good medical practice which is contained by relatively clear legal and moral guidelines'.[11]

The basic position in American law is similar to that of English law, i.e. the humanitarian motive of the physician in seeking to relieve pain and suffering is not a defence to a charge of murder.[12] As already observed, questions relating to the termination of the lives of the critically ill are treated to a much greater extent in statute and case law in the USA than they are in England. Before proceeding to a detailed outline of the principles enunciated by American courts in the context of terminating life-saving treatment, it is worthwhile noting that the active role of the legislature and judiciary of the USA in this area is not necessarily the best way of resolving the problems of the treatment of the critically ill. One example from the statute book and another from the case law ought to suffice for this point to be made in the context of the present brief excursus.

One of the best-known pieces of legislation in this area is the Californian Natural Death Act, 1976. Under this Act, life-sustaining procedures may be withheld from a critically ill patient if he signs a directive to his physicians to this effect. the Act itself, however, contains limitations with regard to the factors the physician may take into account in considering whether or not the patient is indeed in a terminal, incurable, condition, and key terms such as 'artificial means to sustain', and 'when death is imminent' are left undefined.[13] In the light of these observations, it has been suggested that the California Act is in fact too restrictive and may, in the final analysis, act as a smokescreen for the real problems of the dying patient.[14]

In the case of *Re Storar* (1981) 438 NYS 2d 266, the court attempted to deal with the definition of extraordinary treatment, but the main thrust was to distinguish between cases where the incompetent patient has expressed an opinion in health, and those where he had not. It is arguable that such a decision effectively prohibits any physicians from making a decision regarding the patient's treatment which might result in death unless the patient has previously indicated his opinion on the matter. Clearly, such a result can only add confusion to an already sensitive area of medical practice.[15]

The American cases have, however, produced a rich yield of principles and directives in cases involving the termination of life-saving treatment.[16] These include the principle enunciated in *Re Quinlan* (1976) 70 N.J. 355 A 2d 651 that where there is no medical likelihood that a patient in a long-term coma will return to a conscious, cognitive state with continued life-support therapy, there should be no legal obligation to continue such therapy. In *Re Dinnerstein* (1978) 380 NE 2d 134, it was held that where the patient is not in a persistent vegetative state, but is suffering from an incurable disease as a result of which death is imminent, and continued life-support treatment will only briefly prolong the process of dying, then such treatment may be withdrawn. There are, however, no clear guidelines as yet as to whether 'care' such as nourishment and hygiene may also be withdrawn when medical treatment such as artificial respiration is terminated. Much emphasis is also placed on the wishes of the patient or his family and the opinions of independent physicians. In this context, it is noteworthy that several decisions have emphasised the need for ethics committees which would consider diagnoses in difficult cases. [17] In this respect, at any rate, it is apparent that in the USA, too, the need to remove decisions in this area from the formal court setting to a more informal one is recognised and appreciated.

Notes

1. See ch. 3, third section; and G. Williams, *Textbook of Criminal Law* (London, 1978), p.532.
2. H. Palmer, 'Dr. Adam's trial for murder', *Criminal Law Review* [1957], p.365.
3. *Declaration on Euthanasia (1980)* of the Sacred Congregation for the Doctrine of the Faith; and D. Coggan, 'On dying and dying well', *Proceedings of the Royal Society of Medicine* 70 (1977), 75.
4. *The Times,* 6 November 1981.
5. J. Mason and R. McCall-Smith, *Law and Medical Ethics* (London, 1983), p.179.
6. See Williams, *op. cit.,* p.533.
7. D. Coggan, 'On dying and dying well', *Proceedings of the Royal Society of Medicine* 70 (1977), 73.
8. *R.* v. *Malcharek, R.* v *Steel* [1981] 2 AER 422.
9. See Mason and McCall-Smith, *op. cit.,* p.189.
10. See G. Williams, 'Euthanasia', *Medico-Legal Journal* 41 (1973), 14; I. Kennedy, 'Switching off life support machines: the legal implications', *Criminal Law Review* (1977), 443.
11. Mason and McCall-Smith, *op. cit.,* p.188.
12. *People* v. *Dessauer* (1952) 38 Cal 2d 547; *People* v. *Conley* (1966) 64 Cal 2d 310; *Re Eichner* (1981) 420 NE 2d 64; D. Meyers, *Medico-Legal Implications of Death and Dying* (New York, 1981), p.124.
13. See Meyers, *ibid.,* 492.
14. M. Lappe, 'Dying while living: a critique of allowing-to-die legislation', *Journal of Medical Ethics* 4 (1978), 195.
15. Mason and McCall-Smith, *op. cit.,* p.189.
16. Meyers, *op. cit.,* p.379.
17. See Meyers, *op. cit.,* p.383.

LIST OF POST-TALMUDIC SOURCES

1. *Commentaries on the Mishnah*
   Maimonides's Commentary on the Mishnah (R. Moses b. Maimon 1135-1204)
   Tiferet Yisrael (R. Israel Lipschutz 1782-1861)
   Tosafot Yom Tov (R. Yom Tov Lippman Heller 1579-1654)

2. *Commentaries on the Talmud*
   Meiri (R. Menahem Meiri 1294-1315)
   Ramban (R. Moses b. Nahman 1194-1270)
   Ran (R. Nissim Gerondi 1310-1375)
   Rashba (R. Solomon ibn Adreth 1235-1310)
   Rashi (R. Solomon b. Isaac 1040-1105)
   Ritva (R. Yom Tov Ishvilli 1255-1330)
   Shittah Mekubezet (R. Bezalel Ashkenazi 1520-1593)
   Tosafot (11th-13th centuries)
   Yad Remah (R. Meir Abulafiah 1170-1244)

3. *Mishneh Torah and Supercommentaries*
   Mishneh Torah (R. Moses b. Maimon)
   Hiddushei R. Hayyim Halevi (R. Hayyim Soloveitchik 1853-1918)
   Kesef Mishneh (R. Joseph Karo 1488-1575)
   Maggid Mishneh (R. Vidal of Tolosa 14th century)
   Mishneh Lemelekh (R. Judah Rosanes 1657-1727)
   Or Sameah (R. Meir Simha Hakohen 1843-1926)
   Radbaz (R. David b. Zimra 1479-1573)

4. *Tur and Supercommentaries*
   Tur (R. Jacob b. Asher 1270-1340)
   Bah (R. Joel Sirkes 1561-1640)
   Derishah and Perishah (R. Joseph Falk Katz 1555-1614)

5. *Shulhan Arukh and Supercommentaries*
   Shulhan Arukh (R. Joseph Karo 1488-1575)
   Beth Lehem Yehuda (R. Judah Ayash d. 1760)
   Beth Shmuel (R. Samuel b. Uri 17th century)
   Biur Halakhah (R. Israel Meir Hakohen 1838-1933)
   Divrei Saul (R. Joseph Saul Nathanson 1810-1875)
   Hagahot Hagra (R. Elijah of Vilna 1720-1797)
   Magen Avraham (R. Abraham Gumbiner 1637-1683)
   Pithei Teshuva (R. Abraham Zvi Eisenstadt 1813-1868)
   Rema (R. Moses Isserless 1530-1572)
   Sema (R. Joshua Falk Katz 1555-1615)
   Siftei Kohen (R. Shabbtai Kohen 1621-1662)
   Taz (R. David Halevi 1586-1667)

6. *Other Halakhic Codes and Compendia*
    Arukh Hashulhan (R. Jehiel Epstein 1829-1908)
    Ha'amek She'elah (R. Naftali Zvi Berlin 1817-1893)
    Hazon Ish (R. Abraham Isaiah Karelitz 1878-1953)
    Hemdat Yisrael (R. Meir Dan Plotzki 1867-1928)
    Korban Netanel (R. Nathaniel Weil 1687-1768)
    Levush Mordekhai (R. Mordekhai Jaffe 1530-1612)
    Mordekhai (R. Mordekhai b. Hillel d. 1298)
    Petah Hadevir (R. Hayyim Pontremoli 17th century)
    Sefer Ha'eshkol (R. Abraham b. Isaac 1110-1179)
    Sefer Haravan (R. Eliezer b. Nathan 1090-1170)
    Sefer Hasidim (R. Judah the Pious d. 1217)
    Sheirei Knesset Hagedolah (R. Hayyim Benveniste 1603-1673)
    Shevet Miyehuda (R. Isser Yehuda Unterman 1886-1976)
    Shiltei Hagiborim (R. Joshua Boaz 16th century)
    Torat Ha'aden (R. Moses b. Nahman)

7. *Responsa*
    Ahiezer (R. Hayyim Ozer Grodzinski 1863-1940)
    Besamim Rosh (R. Saul Berlin 1740-1794; attributed to the Rosh and his circle)
    Beth Avi (R. Isaac Leibes-pub. N.Y. 1976)
    Beth Yitzhak (R. Isaac Schmelkes 1828-1906)
    Emunat Shmuel (R. Aaron Kaidanower 1614-1676)
    Ginat Veradim (R. Abraham b. Mordekhai 17th century)
    Hatam Sofer (R. Moses Sofer 1762-1839)
    Havot Yair (R. Jair Bachrach 1638-1702)
    Hayyim Sha'al (R. Hayyim Joseph Azulai 1724-1806)
    Hayyim Veshalom (R. Hayyim Palaggi 1788-1869)
    Hikrei Lev (R. Rafael Hazan 1741-1820)
    Iggrot Moshe (R. Moses Feinstein 1895-1986)
    Koah Shor (R. Isaac Schorr 19th century)
    Lev Aryeh (R. Aryeh Grossnass-pub. London, 1973)
    Maggid Mereshit (R. Hayyim Alfandri 1660-1733)
    Mahaneh Hayyim (R. Hayyim Sofer 1821-1886)
    Maharam Alashkar (R. Moses Alashkar 1466-1521)
    Maharam Shick (R. Moses Schick 1807-1879)
    Maharaz Hayyes (R. Zvi Hirsh Hayyes 1805-1855)
    Maharit (R. Joseph Trani 1568-1693)
    Melamed Leho'il (R. David Hoffman 1843-1921)
    Migei Haharigah (R. Simon Efrati-pub. Jerusalem, 1961)
    Mishpat Kohen (R. Abraham Isaac Hakohen Kook 1865-1935)
    Mishpetei Uziel (R. Benzion Hai Uziel 1880-1953)
    Nezer Matai (R. Nathan Freidman-pub. Tel-Aviv, 1957)
    Noda Beyehuda (R. Ezekiel Landau 1713-1793)
    Panim Meirot (R. Meir Eisenstadt 1670-1744)
    Radbaz (R. David b. Zimra)
    Rashbash (R. Solomon b. Simon Duran 1400-1467)
    Rav Pa'alim (R. Joseph Hayyim b. Elijah 1835-1909)
    Seridei Esh (R. Jehiel Jacob Weinberg 1885-1966)
    She'elat Ya'avetz (R. Jacob Emden 1697-1776)
    Temim Deim (R. Abraham b. David of Poisqieres 1125-1198)
    Torat Hesed (R. Schneour Zalman of Lublin 1831-1902)
    Yabia Omer (R. Ovadiah Yosef b. 1920)
    Ziz Eliezer (R. Eliezer Judah Waldenburgh b. 1917)
    Zofnat Paneah (R. Joseph Rosen 1858-1936)

8. *Commentaries on the Bible*
    Abrabanel (R. Isaac Abrabanel 1437-1508)
    Beth Haotsar (R. Joseph Engel 1859-1920)
    Malbim (R. Meir Leib Malbim 1809-1879)
    Meshekh Hokhmah (R. Meir Simha Hakohen)
    Ramban (R. Moses b. Nahman)
    Torah Shelemah (R. Menahem Kasher 1895-1985)
    Torah Temimah (R. Barukh Halevi Epstein 1860-1942)

9. *Jewish Thought*
    Derashat Haran (R. Missim Gerondi)
    Guide for the Perplexed (R. Moses b. Maimon)
    Iggrot Rayah (R. Abraham Isaac Hakohen Kook)
    Milhemet Mitzva (R. Solomon b. Simon Duran 1400-1467)
    Sefer Ikkarim (R. Joseph Albo 15th century)
    Treatise on Logic (R. Moses b. Maimon)

10. *Reference Works*
    Arukh Hashalem (R. Nathan of Rome 1035-1110)
    Encyclopaedia Talmudit (ed. R. Meir Bar-Ilan and R. Solomon Zevin)
    Sede Hemed (R. Hayyim Hezekiah Medini 1831-1904)

BIBLIOGRAPHY

Albeck, S., '*Gerama* and *Garme*' in *The Principles of Jewish Law* (ed. M. Elon, Jerusalem, 1975)

Alexander, L., 'Medical Science Under Dictatorship', *New England Journal of Medicine* 241 (1949)

Alon, G., *Mehkarim Betoldot Yisrael* (Tel Aviv, 5727)

Aptowitzer, V., 'The Status of the Embryo in Jewish Law', *Jewish Quarterly Review* n.s. 15 (1924)

Aries, P., *Western Attitudes Towards Death From the Middle Ages to the Present* (Baltimore, 1974)

Atlas, S., *Netivim Bemishpat Ivri* (N.Y., 5738)

Avraham, A., 'Treating the *Goses* and Determining Death' (Heb.), *Sefer Assia* 3 (ed. A. Steinberg, Jerusalem, 5737)

Baer, I., 'The Religious Social Tendency of *Sefer Hasidim*' (Heb.), *Zion* 3 (5698)

Baron, C., 'Medical Paternalism and the Role of Law', *American Journal of Law and Medicine* 4 (1979) 337.

Barth, K., *Church Dogmatics* 3 (Edinburgh, 1961)

Benamozegh, E., *Israel et L'Humanite* (Paris, 1914)

Benyon, H., 'Doctors or Murderers', *Criminal Law Review* (1982)

Ben-Zimra, E., 'Bloodshed by Necessity in Jewish and Israeli Law' (Heb.), *Shenaton Hamishpat Haivri* 3-4 (5736-5737)

Ben-Zimra, E., 'Halakhic Decisions Relating to the Sanctity of Life and Martyrdom in the Holocaust Period' (Heb.), *Sinai* 80 (5737)

Berman, S., 'Noahide Laws' in *The Principles of Jewish Law* (ed. M. Elon, Jerusalem, 1975)

Bleich, J., 'Ethico-Halakhic Consideration in the Practice of Medicine', *Dine Israel* 7 (1976)

Bleich, J., *Contemporary Halakhic Problems* 1 (N.Y., 1977)

Bleich, J., *Contemporary Halakhic Problems* 2 (N.Y., 1983)

Bleich, J., 'The Quinlan Case: A Jewish Prespective' in *Jewish Bioethics* (ed. J. Bleich and F. Rosner, N.Y., 1979)

Blidstein, J., *Ikkronot Mediniim Bemishnat Harambam* (Bar-Ilan, 5743)

Burt, R., 'Authorizing Death of Anomalous Newborns' in *Genetics and the Law* (ed. A. Milansky and G. Annas, N.Y., 1975)

Callahan, D., 'The Sanctity of Life' in *Updating Life and Death*
(ed. D. Cutler, Boston, 1968)

Callahan, D., 'Bioethics as a Discipline' in *Biomedical Ethics and the Law*
(ed. J. Humber and R. Almeder, N.Y., 1977)

Cahana, J., 'The Practice of Medicine in Post-Talmudic Halakhic Literature'
(Heb.), *Sinai* 27 (5710)

Cardozo, B., *Law and Literature and Other Essays and Addresses* (N.Y., 1931)

Cohen, B., *Jewish and Roman Law* 2 (N.Y., 1966)

Cohen, J., '*Dina Demalkhuta* and the Improvement of Society' (Heb.),
Hatorah Vehamedinah 1 (5709)

Cohn, H., 'The Secularization of Jewish Law' in *Jewish Law in Ancient and
Modern Israel* (ed. H. Cohn, N.Y., 1971)

Cohn, H., 'Divine Punishment' in *The Principles of Jewish Law* (ed. M. Elon,
Jerusalem, 1975)

Cohn, H., 'On the Dichotomy of Divinity and Humanity in Jewish Law' in
Euthanasia (ed. a. Carmi, Berlin, 1984

Coulson, N., *A History of Islamic Law* (Edinburgh, 1964)

Curran, W., 'The Saikewicz Decision', *New England Journal of Medicine*
270 (1978)

Dagi, A., 'The Paradox of Euthanasia', *Judaism* 23 (1975)

Dan, J., *Torat Hasod Shel Hasidei Ashkenaz* (Jerusalem, 5726)

Daube, D., *Collaboration with Tyranny in Rabbinic Law* (London, 1695)

Dawidowicz, L., *The War Against the Jews* 1933-1945 (N.Y., 1975)

Dorff, E., The Interaction of Jewish Law the Morality', *Judaism* 26 (1977)

Dyck, A., 'Beneficient Euthanasia and Benemortasia: Alternative Views of
Mercy' in *Beneficient Euthanasia* (ed. M. Kohl, N.Y., 1975)

Ellinson, E., 'The Foetus in Jewish Law' (Heb.), *Sinai* 66 (5730)

Elon, M., *Hamishpat Haivri* (Jerusalem, 5733)

Englard, I., The Interaction of Law and Morality in Jewish Law' *Jewish Law
Annual* 6 (forthcoming)

Enker, A., 'Homicide Committed in Circumstances of Duress and Necessity in
Jewish Law' (Heb.), *Shenaton Hamishpat Haivri* 2 (5735)

Enker, A., *Hekhrah Vezorekh Bedinei Onshin* (Bar-Ilan, 5737)

Erusi, R. 'Abortion: Theory and Practice in the Halakhah' (Heb.), *Dine Israel*
8 (5737)

Faur, J., *Iyunim Bemishneh Torah: Sefer Hamada* (Jerusalem, 5738)

Federbush, S., *Hamusar Vehamishpat Beyisrael* (Jerusalem, 5739)

Feinstein, M., 'On the Law Concerning the Killing of a Foetus' (Heb.), *R. Ezekiel
Abramski Memorial Volume* (ed. M. Hirshler, Jerusalem 5735)

Finnis, J. *Natural Law and Natural Rights* (Oxford, 1980)

Fletcher, J., 'Ethics and Euthanasia', in *To Live and To Die* (ed. R. Williams,
N.Y., 1973)

Fogelman, M., 'Practical *Halakhah* and Concealed *Halakhah*' (Heb.), *Hatsofeh
Lehokhmat Yisrael* 15 (5691)

Fox, M., 'Maimonides and Aquinas on Natural Law', *Dine Israel* 5 (1972)

Freehof, S., *Reform Responsa* (N.Y., 1973)

Fuller, L., The Speluncean Explorers', *Harvard Law Review* 62 (1948-1949)

Gershuni, J., 'The Law of the *Sanhedrin* and the Monarchy and the Difference Between Them' (Heb.), *Hatorah Vehamedinah* 2 (5710)

Gershuni, J., *Mishpat Hamelukhah* (Jerusalem, 5740)

Gershuni, J., *Kol Zafayikh* (Jerusalem, 5740)

Ginzburg, J., *Mishpatim Leyisrael* (Jerusalem, 5716)

Glazebrook, P., 'The Necessity Plea in English Common Law', *Cambridge Law Journal* (1972a)

Glover, J., *Causing Death and Saving Lives* (Penguin, 1981)

Goldman, E., 'Morality, Religion and *Halakhah*' (Heb.), *Deot* 20 (5723), 21 (5723)

Grisez, G. and Shaw, R., *Beyond the New Morality: The Responsibility of Freedom* (London, 1974)

Halevi, H., 'Disconnecting a Hopeless Patient From an Artificial Respirator' (Heb.), *Tehumin* 2 (5741)

Halibard, G., 'Euthanasia', *Jewish Law Annual* 2 (1978)

Harris, J., *Legal Philosophies* (London, 1980)

Harris, J., *Violence and Responsibility* (London, 1980)

Hart, H., *The Concept of Law* (Oxford, 1964)

Herzog, I. 'The King's Right to Pardon Convicted Offenders in Jewish Law' (Heb.), *Hatorah Vehamedinah* 1 (5709)

Herzog, I., *The Main Institutions of Jewish Law* (London, 1967)

Hirshler, M. 'The Obligation to Save Life' (Heb.), *Halakhah Urefuah* 2 (5741)

Jackson, B., *Essays in Jewish and Comparative Legal History* (Leiden, 1975)

Jackson, B., 'The Concept of Religious Law in Judaism', *Aufsteig und Niedergang der Romischen Welt* 19 (1979)

Jakobowitz, I., 'Concerning the Possibility of Permitting the Precipitation of the Death of a Fatally Ill Patient in Severe Pain' (Heb.), *Hapardes* 31 (5717)

Jakobowitz, I., *Harefuah Vehayahadut* (Jerusalem, 5726)

Kamisar, Y., 'Some Non-Religious Views Against Proposed Mercy-Killing Legislation: A Rejoinder' in *Death, Dying and Euthanasia* (ed. D. Horan and D. Mall, Maryland, 1980)

Katz, E., 'Regarding the Issue of Disconnecting a Fatally Ill Patient from an Artificial Respirator' (Heb.), *Tehumin* 3 (5742)

Katz, J., *Exclusiveness and Tolerance* (N.Y., 1972)

Kennedy, I., 'Switching Off Life-Support Machines: The Legal Implications', *Criminal Law Journal* (1977)

Keyserlingk, E., *Sanctity of Life or Quality of Life* (Ottowa, 1979)

Kohl, M. 'Voluntary Beneficent Euthanasia' in *Beneficient Euthanasia* (ed. M. Kohl, N.Y., 1975)

Kook, S., 'Killing a Suffering Individual' (Heb.), *Torah Shebal Peh* 18 (5736)

Lamm, N. and Kirschenbaum, A., 'Freedom and Constraint in the Judicial Process', *Cardozo Law Review* (1979)

Leibowitz, I., *Medicine and the Value of Human Life: Meshin Inaugural Lecture in the History of Medicine* (Tel Aviv, 1977)

Lerner, R., 'Natural Law in Albo's *Book of Roots*' in *Ancients and Moderns* (ed. J. Cropsey, N.Y., 1964)

Levi, I., 'An Impediment to the Emergence of the Soul' *(Heb.), Noam* 16 (5733)

Lichtenstein, A., 'Does Jewish Tradition Recognize an Ethic Independent of Halakhah?' in *Contemporary Jewish Ethics* (ed. M. Kellner, N.Y., 1978)

Lifshitz, B. 'The Legal Status of the *Responsa* Literature' (Heb.), *Shenaton Hamishpat Haivri* 9-10 (5742-5743)

Lloyd, D. and Freeman, M., *Lloyd's Introduction to Jurisprudence* (London, 1985)

Louisell, D., 'Euthanasia and Biathanasia: On Dying and Killing' in *Death, Dying and Euthanasia* (ed. D. Horan and D. Mall, Maryland, 1980)

MacCormick, N., *Legal Reasoning and Legal Theory* (Oxford, 1978)

Mason, K. and McCall Smith, R., *Law and Medical Ethics* (London, 1983)

Meyers, D., *Medico-Legal Implications of Death and Dying* (N.Y., 1981)

Novak, D., *The Image of the Non-Jew in Judaism* (N.Y., 1983)

Potolsky, M. 'The Rabbinic Rule 'No Laws are Derived from Before Sinai'' (Heb.), *Dine Israel* (5736)

Quint, E. and Hecht, N. *Jewish Jurisprudence* (N.Y., 1980)

Rabinowitz, B., 'A Symposium on the Determination of Death and Organ Transplantation' (Heb.), *Sefer Assia* (ed. A. Steinberg, Jerusalem, 5739)

Rabinowitz, G., 'The Treatment of the Critically Ill, the *Goses,* and the Definition of Death' (Heb.), *Halakhah Urefuah* 1 (5738)

Rachels, J., 'Active and Passive Euthanasia', *New England Journal of Medicine* 292 (1975)

Ramsey, P. *The Patient as Person* (New Haven, 1970)

Ramsey, P. 'The Morality of Abortion' in *Moral Problems: A Collection of Philosophical Essays* (ed. J. Rachels, N.Y., 1971)

Relman, A., 'The Saikewicz Decision: Judges As Physicians'', *New England Journal of Medicine* 270 (1978)

Rosenbaum, I., *The Holocaust and Halakhah* (N.Y., 1976)

Rosenthal, E., 'Some Aspects of Islamic Political Thought', *Islamic Culture* 22 (1948)

Rosner, F., 'Organ Transplantation in Jewish Law' in *Jewish Bioethics* (ed. J. Bleich and F. Rosner, N.Y., 1979)

St. John Stevas, N. *The Right of Life* (N.Y., 1964)

Schacht, J., 'The Law' in *Unity and Variety in Muslim Civilization* (ed. G. von Grunebaugm, Chicago, 1955)

Scholem, G., *Major Trends in Jewish Mysticism* (N.Y., 1940)

Schwarzchild, S., 'Do Noachites Have to Believe in Revelation?' *Jewish Quarterly Review* n.s. 52 (1962)

Sereni, G., *Into that Darkness: From Mercy-Killing to Mass Murder* (London, 1974)

Shilo, S., *Dina Demalkhuta Dina* (Jerusalem, 5735)

Shilo, S., 'Sacrificing One Life for the Sake of Saving Many Lives' (Heb.), *Hevra Vehistoria* (Jerusalem, 5740)

Shilo, S., 'Rejecting One Life for the Sake of Saving Another' (Heb.), *Emunah Beshoah* (Jerusalem, 5740)

Simpson, A., '*Regina* v. *Archer and Muller* (1875): The Leading Case that Never Was', *Oxford Journal of Legal Studies* 2 (1982)

Simpson A., *Cannibalism and the Common Law* (Chicago, 1984)

Smith, J. and Hogan, D., *Criminal Law* (London, 1982)

Soloveitchik, H. ' Three Themes in Sefer Hasidim', *Association for Jewish Studies Review* 1 (1976)

Steinberg, A., 'Mercy-Killing in the Light of the *Halakhah*' Heb.), *Sefer Assia* 3 (ed. A. Steinberg, Jerusalem, 5743)

Stern, M., *Harefuah Leor Hahalakhah* 1 (Jerusalem, 5740)

Taurek, J., 'Should the Numbers Count?', *Philosophy and Public Affairs* 6 (1977)

Telushkin, N., 'The Authority of Man Over his Own Life in the Light of *Halakhah*' *(Heb.), Or Hamizrah* 8 (5721)

Teumim-Rabinowitz, B., 'Capital Offences under the Law of the *Sanhedrin* and of the King Respectively' (Heb.), *Hatorah Vehamedinah* 4 (5712)

Teumim-Rabinowitz, B., 'Extradition to Non-Jewish Authorities' (Heb.), *Noam* 17 (5734)

Trachtenberg, J., *Jewish Magic and Superstition* (N.Y., 1939)

Twersky, I., *Introduction to the Code of Maimonides* (New Haven, 1980)

Veatch, R., *Death, Dying and the Biological Revolution* (New Haven, 1976)

Walton, D., *On Defining Death* (Montreal, 1979)

Warhaftig, I., 'Self-Defence in the Crimes of Homicide and Assault' (Heb.), *Sinai* 81 (5737)

Weinberger, J., 'Mercy-Killing in Jewish Law in the Light of the *Halakhah*' *(Heb.), Dine Israel* 7 (5737)

Weinfeld, M., 'The Genuine Jewish Attitude Towards Abortion" (Heb.), *Zion* 42 (5737)

Weiss, I., *Dor Dor Vedorshav* (Berlin, 1923)

Werner, S., 'Mercy-Killing in the Light of Jewish Law' (Heb.), *Torah Shebal Peh* 18 (5736)

Williams, G., 'Euthanasia', *Medico-Legal Journal* 14 (1973)

Williams, G., *Textbook of Criminal Law* (London, 1983)

Wisebard, A. 'On the Bioethics of Jewish Law: The Case of Karen Quinlan', *Israel Law Review* 14 (1979)

Wolner, M., 'The Physician's Rights and Jurisdiction' (Heb.), *Hatorah Vehamedinah* 7-8 (5716-5717)

112   Bibliography

Yisraeli, S., 'The Authority of the President and Elected Governmental
    Institutions in the State of Israel' (Heb.), *Hatorah Vehamedinah* 1 (5709)

Yisraeli, S., 'The Legal Jurisdiction of the Monarchy in Contemporary Times'
    (Heb.), *Hatorah Vehamedinah* 2 (5710)

Zweig, M. 'Concerning Abortion' (Heb.), *Noam* 7 (5724)

TABLE OF ENGLISH AND AMERICAN CASES

INDEX